Bolden and Takle's
PRACTICE NURSE HANDBOOK

Other books of interest:

The Royal Marsden Hospital Manual of Clinical Nursing Procedures
Third edition
A. Phylip Pritchard and Jane Mallett
0 632 03387 8

Health Promotion – Concepts and Practice
A. Dines and A. Cribb
0 632 03543 9

Expanding the Role of the Nurse – The Scope of Professional Practice
G. Hunt and P. Wainwright
0 632 03604 4

Practice Management
Second edition
K. J. Bolden, A. P. Lewis and B. Sawyer
0 632 03319 3

Blackwell's Dictionary of Nursing
0 632 03808 X Hardback
0 632 03561 7 Paperback

Managing Asthma in Primary Care
A. Crockett
0 632 03757 1

A Practical Guide to Fundholding
R. Smith, S. Brogan, N. Ralph and R. Stephenson
0 632 03869 1

Bolden and Takle's
PRACTICE NURSE HANDBOOK

Third Edition

GILLIAN D HAMPSON

RGN, RCNT, Dip in Nursing (Lond)
DN Cert PWT, FPCert
Practice Nurse, Chartfield Surgery, Putney
Practice Nurse Trainer, Kingston and Richmond FHSA

BLACKWELL SCIENTIFIC PUBLICATIONS

OXFORD LONDON EDINBURGH BOSTON

MELBOURNE PARIS BERLIN VIENNA

© 1984, 1989, 1994 by
Blackwell Scientific Publications
Editorial Offices:
Osney Mead, Oxford OX2 0EL
25 John Street, London WC1N 2BL
23 Ainslie Place, Edinburgh EH3 6AJ
238 Main Street, Cambridge,
  Massachusetts 02142, USA
54 University Street, Carlton,
  Victoria 3053, Australia

Other Editorial Offices:
Librairie Arnette SA
1, rue de Lille
75007 Paris
France

Blackwell Wissenschafts-Verlag GmbH
Kurfürstendamm 57
10707 Berlin
Germany

Blackwell MZV
Feldgasse 13
A-1238 Wien
Austria

First Edition published 1984
Second Edition published 1989
Reprinted 1989
Third Edition published 1994

Set by DP Photosetting, Aylesbury, Bucks
Printed and bound in Great Britain by
Bell and Bain, Ltd, Glasgow

DISTRIBUTORS

Marston Book Services Ltd
PO Box 87
Oxford OX2 0DT
(*Orders:* Tel: 0865 791155
         Fax: 0865 791927
         Telex: 837515)

USA
Blackwell Scientific Publications, Inc.
238 Main Street
Cambridge, MA 02142
(*Orders:* Tel: 800 759-6102
         617 876 7000)

Canada
Oxford University Press
70 Wynford Drive
Don Mills
Ontario M3C 1J9
(*Orders:* Tel: (416) 441-2941)

Australia
Blackwell Scientific Publications Pty Ltd
54 University Street
Carlton, Victoria 3053
(*Orders:* Tel: 03 347-5552)

A catalogue record for this book is available
from the British Library

ISBN 0–632–03692–3

Library of Congress
Cataloging in Publication Data
Hampson, Gillian D.
    Bolden and Takle's Practice nurse
handbook. — 3rd ed./Gillian D. Hampson.
    p.   cm.
    Rev. ed. of: Practice nurse handbook/
Keith J. Bolden, Beryl A. Takle, 2nd ed.
1989.
    Includes bibliographic references and
index.
    ISBN 0-632-03692-3
    1. Nurse practitioners.   2. Primary
care (Medicine)   3. Nurse
practitioners—Great Britain.   I. Bolden,
Keith J. Practice nurse handbook.
II. Takle, Beryl A.   III. Title.   IV. Title:
Practice nurse handbook.
    [DNLM: 1. Nursing. 2. Family Practice.
WY 101 H231b 1994]
RT82.8.H35   1994
610.73′06′92—dc20
DNLM/DLC
for Library of Congress   94-5301
                                        CIP

Contents

Foreword to the First Edition

The past ten years have seen a steady growth in the number of nurses employed by general practitioners to work in surgery treatment rooms. The wide range of skills required of nurses undertaking such work effectively prompted the Steering Group, established to consider 'The Training Needs of the Practice Nurse', to recommend that these nurses should in future receive recognised training for their role.

This book is, therefore, a welcome and timely publication, not just for the new recruit to practice nursing, but for the established practice nurse intent upon developing the role further, particularly in the field of anticipatory care as considered in the Royal College of General Practitioners Report 'Promoting Prevention'.

The book covers the whole range of knowledge and skills required by a practice nurse during the course of the day-to-day activities in a treatment room. In addition to containing useful chapters on the organisation of general practice and the nurse and the law it offers a very practical guide on equipping a treatment room. A great strength of the book for many practice nurses will be the chapters on nursing procedures, not only because of the attention to detail but for the variety of procedures particularly relevant to the general practice setting which are included.

The clear exposition of the role and function of the practice nurse should enhance professional awareness of the contribution which a nurse makes within the setting of general practice, as should acknowledgement of the part played by the practice nurse alongside that of general practitioner, district nurse and health visitor colleagues within the primary health care team.

Keith Bolden and Beryl Takle, the authors, write with knowledge and understanding of practice nurses and their training needs. This book is published at an opportune moment and should become essential reading, both as a textbook for those in training and a reference book for those already in practice. It should find a place on the shelves of nursing libraries and become a standard text for use by practice nurses.

Annia Fawcett-Henesy

Preface to the Second Edition

Since this book was first written five years ago there have been tremendous developments in both the clinical and medico-political fields for practice nurses. Their role is now well established and this book has been revised and rewritten to take account of the many exciting changes which have occurred and to look at the present areas of development.

We hope that those attending training courses for practice nurses will find this book particularly helpful.

Keith J. Bolden
Beryl A. Takle

Preface to the Third Edition

This book has been the mainstay for thousands of us since we quitted the familiar territory of the NHS for the uncharted waters of nursing in general practice. Phenomenal changes within nursing and the health service have made revision of the book imperative, but rewriting the work of my mentors has been no easy task. There was so much new material to incorporate that difficult choices had to be made over what to leave out. I kept three objectives before me: to give as many practical hints and pointers as possible, to draw attention to the legal pitfalls awaiting the unwary, and finally, to point out ways in which practice nurses can develop their role.

I trust that this edition will be as useful to practice nurses as the previous editions have been.

Gillian D. Hampson

Acknowledgements

Four people deserve special thanks for their help while I was writing this edition: my husband Peter who did all the household chores, my colleague Faith Lewis who did more than her share of the work in our practice, Caroline Fox who edited some of my notes, and Peter Rosenfelder who helped with the word processing and graphics. Thanks are also due to my employers Drs John Dymond and Jennifer Lebus, and to the people too numerous to mention, who generously gave me advice and information on their special subjects.

Chapter 1
Teamwork in General Practice

This first chapter outlines the background to the work of practice nurses so that the role can be considered within the context of the whole primary health care team.

The National Health Service (NHS)

In 1948 the National Health Service was established on the basis that everybody should have free access to medical care irrespective of their financial state. It seems naive now to realise that it was assumed the demand for care would decrease once the unresolved 'pool' of illness in the population had been treated. In the light of experience it has become clear that the amount of treatable illness is small, compared with either chronic conditions which cannot be cured, or the problems created by environmental and personal stress (the underlying reasons for many consultations in general practice).

Developments in general practice

Prior to 1948 most general practitioners worked independently, usually from their own homes[1]. Patients who were unable to afford private medical care belonged to a doctor's 'panel'. The cost was supported by various insurance schemes, and hospital beds were endowed especially for 'the poor'. The hospitals were nationalised in 1948 but general practitioners, dentists, retail pharmacists and opticians stayed as independent businesses with contracts to supply specific services to NHS patients. Executive Councils were set up to administer these arrangements. Other services, such as district nursing and health visiting were under the control of local authorities.

The early days of the NHS were a catalogue of disasters with neither doctors nor patients really knowing what to expect of the new system. Patients had been led to believe that everything was 'free'; so extra demands were made upon doctors who were themselves unprepared for the organisational and practical difficulties created by the new system. Between 1948 and 1956 expenditure in the NHS had risen by 70%[2].

'The GPs' Charter'

The British Medical Association, through its General Medical Services Committee, has always been responsible for the political aspects of general practice. This includes terms of service and remuneration. The College of General Practitioners, established in 1953 (to become the Royal College in 1966), was more concerned with the educational aspects of practice. The effects of these two bodies on government policies brought about in 1966 the so-called 'GPs' Charter', in response to the threat of resignation by disillusioned doctors[3]. The 'charter' radically altered the way in which GPs were paid, and gave them incentives for having better premises and more staff.

Vocational training

Postgraduate training for general practice was introduced on a more formal basis in 1973; followed by the Vocational Training Act in 1981. It is now impossible to become a principal in general practice without three years specific postgraduate training, which includes one year as a trainee in an approved practice.

The development and recognition of general practice as a specialty in its own right has been compared with the similar difficulties faced by practice nurses within their own profession[4].

NHS reorganisation

The structure of the NHS was reorganised in 1974, when 'management' first assumed a specialist function[5]. Executive Councils became Family Practitioner Committees (FPCs), and community nurse employment was transferred from local authorities to the health service.

Area Health Authorities were abolished in 1982 and their powers devolved to District Health Authorities (DHAs)[6]. However, 1990 saw the most radical changes yet to the NHS. The introduction of the internal market created a separation between the purchasers and the providers of services. Hospitals were invited to become self-governing trusts; individual departments could become provider units and negotiate their own contracts and GPs in large group practices were encouraged to become fundholders to purchase hospital services on behalf of their patients. FPCs were changed to Family Health Service Authorities (FHSAs) with greater managerial responsibilities in relation to general practice[7].

The structure of the NHS

Although politics can seem remote from direct patient care, it is useful to keep abreast of developments in the way the NHS is organised (Fig. 1.1). The structures for Scotland, Wales and Northern Ireland are all slightly different; the Secretary of State for each of these has overall responsibility for the NHS. Reference to FHSAs is made for convenience throughout this book, although Scotland and Northern Ireland have Health Boards instead.

The NHS Policy Board decides the overall strategy for the National Health Service. The various directorates and branches of the NHS

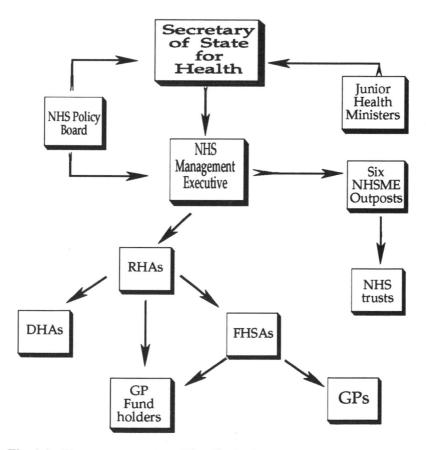

Fig. 1.1 The structure of the NHS in England.

Management Executive (NHSME) are responsible for the operation of the service in terms of effectiveness and value for money.

Community Health Councils (CHCs) represent the consumers of the NHS through members drawn from local authorities, voluntary services and representatives of the local community. CHCs have a right to be consulted about hospital closures and significant changes to the local NHS services but they have no executive powers.

The new GP contract

In 1990 the government imposed a new contract on general practitioners, requiring them to provide a range of screening and health promotion services. Many practice nurses were employed at that time to undertake the extra work[8]. Some GPs were sceptical about the value of many of these activities, which were not supported by scientific proof of their validity[9]. Some aspects of the contract have been modified since then. Apart from the medical services already offered to patients, the new contract required GPs to be responsible for:

- *Child health surveillance* – developmental checks up to the age of five for which a single fee may be claimed.
- *Registration health checks* – for all patients age 5–75. A fee can be claimed.
- *Adult health checks* – to be offered to patients under 75 who had not seen the doctor in the past three years. (This requirement has since been dropped.)
- *Health promotion clinics* – for which fees could be claimed. (Clinic fees were replaced in 1993 by targets payments for specific health promotion activities.)
- *Minor surgery* – by doctors accepted onto the minor surgery list. Fees can be claimed for 15 minor operations a quarter.

The 'Patients' Charter'

In 1992 patients acquired new rights as consumers, through the part of the *Citizens' Charter* relating to the NHS – the *Patients' Charter*[10]. One of the standards includes having a named qualified nurse responsible for a patient's care.

The health of the nation

In that same year, the government introduced targets for reducing disease and disability through its *Health of the Nation* strategy for

England[11]. Examples are given in later chapters. Similar strategies were produced in the other countries of Great Britain.

Care in the community

Other changes accelerated within the community from April 1993 as a result of the NHS and Community Care Act (1990)[12]. Social service departments assumed new responsibilities for assessing the needs and providing tailor-made services for vulnerable people. Hospitals had to ensure that the appropriate services were in place before such patients could be discharged home. More resources were needed to provide effective community care. Proposals were made to close several teaching hospitals in London and to transfer the staff and resources to the community[13].

The changes in the NHS were intended to give:

- *Consumer choice* – through the involvement of patients and voluntary groups in decisions.
- *Value for money* – through effective management.
- *Quality services* – through clinical audit and review.

General practice

All non-private general practitioners have the same contract with the NHS. Unlike hospital doctors, who are salaried, they have a complicated system of remuneration. The *Statement of Fees and Allowances* (known as the *Red Book*) gives details of all the payments which GPs may receive from the NHS[14]. Payments include:

- *Basic practice allowance* – towards the costs incurred in providing medical services to NHS patients.

- *Capitations fees* – for each patient registered. Higher rates are paid for patients over 65 and 75 years of age; to reflect the increased health care needs of older people.
  Additional payments are made to reflect either the increased cost of travelling in rural practices, or the extra work generated in areas of social deprivation (calculated using the Jarman Index of deprivation[15]).

- *Item of service fees* – can be claimed for additional services, e.g. family planning, registration health checks, some immunisation.

(Payments for cervical screening and childhood immunisation are only made when overall targets are reached.) Maternity care, night visits and emergency treatment all attract fees. Special claim forms are needed.

- *Other payments* – ancillary staff salaries and training costs qualify for partial reimbursement. Although 70% reimbursement obtained under the previous system, the FHSAs have greater discretion over the allocation of funds, and consequently can stipulate certain conditions to be met before reimbursement will be made.

Other diverse activities, such as teaching medical students or dispensing, will earn payments. The postgraduate education allowance (PGEA) is paid to doctors who attend the equivalent of five study days a year.

Apart from payments by the NHS, general practitioners are entitled to charge for activities not covered by their Contract such as writing reports, private medical certificates and examinations, or treating private patients.

GP fundholding

Fundholding practices receive funds from the FHSA to cover the practice running costs of staff, premises and equipment. A drugs budget is also fixed to indicate the limits of prescribing, which ideally should not be exceeded.

Regional Health Authorities (RHAs) set budgets for purchasing hospital inpatient and outpatient services and district nursing and health visiting. The functions of the RHAs in England are being devolved to district level[16]. Many FHSAs are combining with district health authorities as purchasing authorities, and some local authorities are expressing an interest in becoming purchasers.

Practice population profiles

The changes within the NHS necessitate the identification of the particular health and social needs of local populations, in order to provide appropriate services. Such profiles should cover: age/sex ratios, ethnic groups, family structures, social class, employment, housing, vulnerable groups, morbidity and mortality, environmental hazards and amenities[17].

Teamwork

The explosion of work within general practice highlights the need for good teamwork, but just being together in one place will not create a team. All teams share certain characteristics, whatever their functions:

- A shared purpose or goal.
- A sense of team identity.
- An understanding of the role, and valuing of the contribution of individual team members.

Teamwork needs some committed hard work to succeed. It can be hindered by ineffective leadership, divided loyalties when members belong to more than one team, or sabotage by disaffected members.

The historical background to the different professions means that nurses trained in a rigidly hierarchical system, and GPs accustomed to assume authority, may have very different perceptions of the same situation. The importance of team building has been recognised for many years in the commercial world and many of their methods are being adopted in the health service. Teambuilding workshops are organised by FHSAs in conjunction with the Health Education Authority's Primary Health Care Unit at Oxford[18].

Primary health care

Primary health care refers to health promotion and care within the community, as compared with secondary care provided by hospitals and specialist services[19]. Primary health care teams have been around since the 1960s in one guise or another, but in reality there are often two types of team involved with general practice.

The practice team

A practice team tends to incorporate all those people based within the practice; most of whom are either partners, or directly employed by the GP. Apart from the doctors, practice teams include:

The practice nurse(s) (see Chapter 2).

The title Practice Nurse has always been generally understood to apply to a qualified nurse employed directly by a general practitioner or GP partnership. Over 90% of practice nurses are Registered General Nurses (RGN), according to the first report of the national census of practice nurses[20].

The practice manager

A practice manager has responsibility for organising the systems which allow the practice to run smoothly and for promoting a high quality service to the patients. The practice manager is also responsible for the financial and personnel management, staff development and liaison with all the staff, the FHSA and other bodies.

The original practice managers were often senior receptionists, for whom this was a logical promotion. However a new breed of practice manager has emerged with the specific management training needed. Many are members of the Association of Health Centre and Practice Administrators. Fundholding practices may also employ separate business managers to deal specifically with the placing of contracts, management of the budget, and monitoring of the services provided.

The receptionist(s)

Receptionists are the first point of contact with the public. They must be able to stay calm in the face of conflicting demands from patients, other staff and the telephone. Receptionists frequently act as 'gate-keepers' to the doctor by prioritising appointments or controlling the number of telephone calls put through. A very fine line exists between efficient organisation and denial of a patient's right to consult the GP.

Apart from running the appointment system and taking telephone messages, there is plenty of administrative work. Many practices are computerised and registration data has to be processed. Some receptionists organise repeat prescriptions and help to complete item of service fee claims. Filing clerks prepare the records for surgery sessions, and file letters, reports and the patients' records after use.

Training for receptionists often takes place 'in-house', but courses are also available. The Practice Receptionist Programme[21], organised by some FHSAs and colleges of further education, leads to a qualification from the Association of Medical Secretaries and Practice Receptionists (AMSPAR).

The medical secretary

A medical secretary needs office skills and a knowledge of the terminology used in medical correspondence. In smaller practices secretarial duties may be combined with reception work, but large practices usually employ a qualified medical secretary to deal with referral letters, reports and the practice correspondence.

Paramedical staff

Larger practices may employ or facilitate other professional staff – dieticians, physiotherapists, counsellors and chiropodists, to increase the range of services available for patients. Pharmacists are joining some practices to help with more effective prescribing. Alternative therapists such as acupuncturists, aromatherapists and masseuses are also being welcomed into some teams.

The primary health care team (PHCT)

The dream that community nurse attachment to GP practices would lead to integrated primary care teams has rarely been realised fully[22]. Even so, group attachment does allow for better communication between the professional groups than when nurses work in geographical patches[23]. District nurses, health visitors, community midwives and community psychiatric nurses also relate to nursing teams in their own specialties, which may have different aims and priorities from those of the practice. Doctors in fundholding practices now negotiate contracts for district nursing and health visiting services, but misunderstandings are still possible. Advice is available for GPs on buying community nursing[24].

In the future, practice nurses may form consortia with other community nurses to market their skills and expertise to the budget-holders. The future of community nursing depends partly on the implementation of the proposals by the United Kingdom Central Council (UKCC) for community education and practice[25]. At present, district nurses and health visitors undertake post-registration courses in their own specialties at institutes of higher education, to equip them for their different roles.

District nurses

A district nurse is responsible for providing skilled nursing services in the community by:

- assessing the care needs of patients and their families,
- formulating individualised care plans and revising them as necessary,

- implementing the care or delegating to other members of the district nursing team,
- monitoring the patients' progress and reassessing care needs.

Liaison with other PHCT members, social services and voluntary agencies is often as important as direct care-giving. The role also includes teaching other nurses, medical students and GP trainees. District nursing teams work in a similar way to hospital ward teams, with mixed skills and grades.

Health visitors

The role of health visitors is in a state of change. Their concerns with public health in the Victorian era led to health visitor involvement with maternal and child welfare. Many health visitors still devote a high proportion of their time to work with the under-fives. However, the role can encompass health promotion (as defined in Chapter 9) with people of all ages, and the importance of the public health role has also been reasserted recently. Health visitors in deprived areas are developing many innovative ways of improving the health and welfare of their clients[26]. As with the district nurses, teaching and liaison with other agencies are important aspects of the role of health visitors.

Health visitors can help to compile a profile of individual practice populations, so that the primary health care team can target services to the groups with particular health needs locally[27].

Community midwives

Community midwives have statutory responsibilities for the care of women during pregnancy, confinement and the puerperium[28]. Community midwives organise antenatal and postnatal care in health centres and general practices, and run antenatal and parentcraft classes. A community midwife must attend a home confinement, and be responsible for a domino scheme or delivery within a GP hospital maternity unit. The midwife will care for a mother and baby until at least the tenth day after delivery, and notify the health visitor when they are discharged.

In remote areas, such as the Scottish islands, one person may hold a triple role as district nurse, midwife and health visitor.

Other nurses

Other nurses may be considered as peripheral members of the PHCT.

Each has a specific contribution to make, but the links with general practice are often more tenuous.

Community psychiatric nurses (CPNs) – are registered mental health nurses, most of whom have completed a post-registration course. The service developed out of hospital-based psychiatric nursing, and most CPNs continue to be based in hospitals. CPNs carry out mental health assessments with patients and their families within the community, and offer a range of therapeutic strategies[29].

Hospital and community-based specialist nurses – are a valuable resource for advice and teaching on their individual subjects – e.g. diabetes, continence, stoma care, HIV/AIDS and infection control.

School nurses – have a major role in health promotion for school children, as well as in dealing with their health problems at school. Practice nurses may have most contact with school nurses through the care of children with asthma.

Social services

Referrals can be made on behalf of patients who require home care, 'meals on wheels' or other social service support. However, few practices have a social worker attached and referrals for social services are usually made by telephone or letter. Social workers are required to make a full needs assessment of the patients referred to them.

Health visitors and GPs are sometimes involved with social workers on child protection issues. An approved social worker is needed when a patient is compulsorily detained under the Mental Health Act (see Chapter 14).

Voluntary services

A huge number of voluntary services, self-help groups and charities exist. They provide financial and practical assistance, as well as information, advice, and research funding. Some are organised locally to help people in need in that community, while others help sufferers of a specific illness or disability.

Patients and their carers can benefit from the knowledge of a practice nurse who can tell them who to approach for help. A database of contact addresses can be built up, either in a manual file or on the computer.

Some practices have a league of friends who organise transport for disabled and immobile patients, arrange prescription collection etc., and sometimes fund raise to buy extra medical equipment for the practice. This type of voluntary work can offer significant help in both urban and rural communities.

Suggestions for evaluation and research

● Compile a diagram of the way the NHS is run within your health district. How are the executive staff appointed?

● Assess the strengths and weaknesses of -
   (a) your practice team
   (b) your primary health care team.
   What changes (if any) could be implemented to improve communication within:
   (a) the practice team?
   (b) the primary health care team?

● What does the health profile of your practice population reveal? Which groups of people need the most help?

● How easy is it to find out about the statutory and voluntary services available locally?

References

1. Stevens, R. (1966) *Medical Practice in Modern England: the Impact of Specialisation and State Medicine.* Yale University Press, USA.
2. Allsop, J. (1984) *Health Policy and the National Health Service.* Longman, Harlow.
3. Ministry of Health (Gillie, A. Chairman) (1963) *The Field of Work of the Family Doctor.* HMSO, London.
4. Bolden, K. and Bolden, S. (1986) Is history repeating itself? *British Medical Journal,* **293:** 19–20.
5. Institute of Health Service Management (1991) *The Hospitals and Health Services Year Book 1991,* 18.62 – 18.70. Institute of Health Service Management, London.
6. Institute of Health Service Management (1991) *The Hospitals and Health Services Year Book 1991,* 18.89–18.95. Institute of Health Service Management, London.

7. Great Britain, Parliament (1990) *The National Health Service and Community Care Act 1990.* HMSO, London.
8. Atkin, K., Lunt, N., Parker, G. and Hirst, M. (1993) *Nurses Count: A National Census of Practice Nurses.* Social Policy Research Unit, University of York.
9. Fry, J. (1990) Health promotion and disease prevention: feasible and worth the effort? *Practice Nurse,* **3:** 257–287.
10. Department of Health (1991) *The Patient's Charter.* DHO, London.
11. Department of Health (1992) *The Health of the Nation: A Strategy for Health in England.* HMSO, London.
12. Great Britain, Parliament (1990) *The National Health Service and Community Care Act 1990.* HMSO, London.
13. Tomlinson, B. (1992) *Report of the Inquiry into London's Health Service. Medical Education and Research.* HMSO, London.
14. DOH, Welsh Office. *Statement of Fees and Allowances to General Medical Practitioners in England and Wales from 1 April 1990.* NHS General Medical Services.
15. Jarman, B. (1983) Identification of underprivileged areas; *British Medical Journal,* **286:** 1705–1709.
16. Department of Health (1993) *Managing the New NHS.* DOH, London.
17. Royal College of Nursing (1993) *The GP Practice Population Profile.* RCN, London.
18. Cook, R. (1992) Workshop solutions dissolve problems; *Practice Nurse,* **5:** 463–466.
19. Report of a working party of the RCN Society of Primary Health Care Nursing (1980) *Primary Health Care Nursing, A Team Approach.* RCN, London.
20. Atkin, K., Lunt, N., Parker, G. and Hirst, M. (1993) *Nurses Count: A National Census of Practice Nurses,* SPRU, University of York.
21. *Practice Receptionist Programme, a Learning Experience for Receptionists.* Radcliffe Medical Press, Oxford.
22. Allsopp, J. (1984) *Health Policy and the National Health Service,* 69–70, Longman, London.
23. Lamb, A. (1977) *Primary Health Nursing.* Bailliere Tindall, London.
24. Royal College of Nursing (1993) *Buying Community Nursing, a Guide for GPs.* RCN, London.
25. United Kingdom Central Council for Nurses, Midwives and Health Visitors (1991) *Report on Proposals for the Future of Community Education and Practice.* UKCC, London.
26. Royal College of Nursing (1994) *Public Health: Nursing Rises to the Challenge.* RCN, London.
27. Royal College of Nursing (1993) *Buying Community Nursing, a Guide for GPs.* RCN, London.
28. UKCC (1993) *Midwives Rules.* UKCC, London.
29. RCN (1993) *Buying Community Nursing, a Guide for GPs.* RCN, London.

Further reading

Poulton, B. and West, M. (1993) Effective Multi-Disciplinary Teamwork in Primary Health Care; *Journal of Advanced Nursing*, June 18: 918–25.
Damant, M., Martin, C. and Openshaw, S. (1994) *Practice Nursing: Stability and Change*. Mosby-Year Book Europe, London.
Adair, J. (1987) *Effective Team-Building*. Pan Books, London.

Useful addresses

HEA Primary Health Care Unit
The Churchill Hospital, Headington, Oxford, OX3 7LJ.

HMSO Publications Centre
PO Box 276, London SW8 5DT.

HMSO Accredited agents (see *Yellow Pages*).

Chapter 2
General Practice Nursing

One of the attractions of practice nursing is the flexibility it allows. Progressive nurses have blossomed in the atmosphere of general practice, and some have become celebrities through their innovation in health promotion and chronic disease management. But herein lies a dilemma: that same flexibility can also lead to a diversity of standards. The revelations in 1993 about unsafe cervical smear techniques reflected the lack of appropriate training and supervision for some staff in general practice[1,2]. In addition many practice nurses have felt themselves to be disadvantaged, in relation to district nurses and health visitors, by the lack of a specific recordable post-basic qualification.

Historical background

Practice nursing developed gradually from the work of GPs' wives who were nurses, and from district nurse attachment to general practice[3]. The Health Services and Public Health Act (1968) gave the seal of approval for district nurses to extend their work to seeing patients in health centres and GP premises. It also legitimised the attachment of nurses to practices, instead of working on a geographical basis[4].

More practice nurses began to be employed by doctors in the early 1970s when it became apparent that the district nurses were unable to spend as long in the surgery, doing tasks like dressings and injections as the doctors were asking them to do. At the same time there were differences of opinion between GPs and the nursing hierarchy about the role of the nurses working in the community. One solution to this was for doctors to employ nurses directly. After 1966, when salaries could be partially reimbursed, practice nurses were classified with secretaries and receptionists as ancillary staff on the Family Practitioner Committee returns. Even as late as 1992, when FHSAs were asked by the Social Policy Research Unit to furnish the names of practice nurses for the National Census, some FHSAs could not identify all the nurses in post[5].

Neighbourhood nursing

The Cumberlege Report in 1986 caused outrage to many practice nurses when it was suggested that all community nurses should be employed in neighbourhood nursing teams[6]. The proposal led to a new sense of group identity as practice nurses came together to fight for the right to continue being employed within general practice[7]. The apparently illogical preference by members of one profession to be employed by members of another, owes much to the negative feelings felt by many practice nurses towards inflexible management in the NHS.

The 'New GP Contract'

The 1990 GP Contract led to a doubling, seemingly overnight, of the number of practice nurses employed[8]. This phenomenon caused a stir in nursing circles and concern at the lack of professional control over such a large group of nurses[9]. Practice nurse education finally began to receive serious attention. (Practice nurse courses had been approved by the National Boards since the joint working party reported on the training needs of practice nurses in 1984[10], but these short courses failed to meet the needs of most nurses[11].)

By 1990 many FHSAs were employing nurse advisers, and/or facilitators who were co-ordinating training. Practice nurses were suddenly overwhelmed by educational opportunities from colleges, FHSAs, specialist societies, drug companies and professional journals. However, there was no simple way of assessing the quality of the education, and the amount of study leave granted to practice nurses varied from practice to practice.

Project 2000

Project 2000 changed the traditional nurse training into a higher education system comparable with that of other disciplines[12]. Initially it was expected that Project 2000 would equip nurses to work in any setting but it became obvious that more education would be needed for work in the community. The United Kingdom Central Council (UKCC) plans for community education and practice will finally give qualified practice nurses and other community nurses equality with district nurses and health visitors as specialist nurses[13]. Practice nurses will have a recordable qualification as General Practice Nurses. Once that happens it remains to be seen how the current employment arrangements for practice nurses will be affected. (The original name is used in this book for the sake of convenience.)

The NHS Management Executive presented another vision – for 'primary health care nursing' in Nursing in Primary Health Care: *New World – New Opportunities*[14].

Practice nurses

The diversity of the work undertaken by practice nurses makes a precise definition of the role very difficult. Instead it can be considered along a continuum:

| Treatment Room | Practice Nurse | Nurse |
| Nurse ◀───▶ | | Practitioner |

Treatment room nurses

Treatment room nurses were originally employed by the health service for nursing work within health centres[15]. They were not employed directly by the general practitioners. 'Treatment room nurse' is often used nowadays to describe a nurse employed to perform specific technical or nursing tasks in the practice. However, up-to-date knowledge and good interpersonal skills are just as essential as manual dexterity, and the role of the treatment room nurse should not be undervalued.

Practice nurses

Practice nurses usually have a wider remit, although nearly all practice nursing contains an element of treatment room work. Practice nursing can be considered under several headings:

Management

- organising the nurses' rooms and work, including call/recall for health promotion,
- maintaining clinical stocks and supplies,
- liaison with the practice manager and GPs on organisational and professional issues, including: policies, protocols and standards of care.

Clinical

- assessing patients' care needs,
- planning, providing, and evaluating the care given, (this includes

technical and nursing procedures as well as screening, and chronic disease management.)

Communication

- giving information, support and advice to patients and carers. Counselling and health promotion,
- liaison with other members of the practice team, the primary health care team, social services and other agencies,
- teaching other nurses and students.

Audit and research

- compiling statistics and reports on nursing activities,
- identifying ways to improve nursing practice.

Because the work of practice nurses is so varied and challenging, it increases the need for up-to-date knowledge. Many practices have a practice library which should include a nursing section. There are many journals relevant to practice nursing (see Appendix 2.1).

Nurse practitioners

Nurse practitioners are very experienced nurses who have had further specialised training at degree level to be able to work autonomously. Diagnostic skills and prescribing, traditionally the prerogative of doctors, are among the subjects taught on nurse practitioner courses.

The term *nurse practitioner* originated in the United States and has its counterpart in many other countries. The first nurse practitioner in the UK (whose background was in health visiting), took up her post in Birmingham in 1982[16]. Since then the numbers have grown considerably. Some nurse practitioners are undertaking outreach work with neglected, underprivileged groups in the community; others have begun working in hospitals and in general practice. Each person has to identify and establish her/his own sphere of influence. Nurse practitioners continue to wait for their own special skills and expertise to be recognised and protected by the UKCC. The issue has not been satisfactorily addressed by the community nursing proposals. Meanwhile there is an overlap with some of the work of practice nurses and the titles are still used rather indiscriminately[17].

Skill-mix

Skill-mix is the name of the system for identifying the knowledge and expertise needed to perform any job, so that the most appropriate person can do it. Nurses in hospitals and the community have become accustomed to skill-mix reviews, but it is relatively new to general practice[18]. Any nurse who wishes to review her/his role can consider each activity in turn and list the knowledge, skills and training needed to perform it effectively. It will become apparent which activities could be delegated, and a case can then be made on economic grounds for utilising nursing skills most effectively.

Nurse employment in general practice

Medical training has traditionally been concerned with diagnosis and treatment, with little time left over for management and personnel matters. It follows that while some GPs are excellent employers, there are others who are less considerate. This can leave an inexperienced nurse vulnerable to exploitation. Even well-meaning GPs have been known to jib at providing contracts of employment, believing them to be unnecessary where there is mutual trust.

The terms and conditions agreed at the interview are binding, but employees who work more than 16 hours a week must have a written contract of employment within 13 weeks of starting work[19]. People who have worked eight or more hours a week for five years are also entitled to a written contract. The law will soon be changed to give part-time workers the same rights as full-time staff.

Nurses accustomed to pay and conditions negotiated by Whitley Councils may never before have had to negotiate on their own behalf. Many nurses are not naturally assertive, so it is important to know what to ask at the interview, and how to present a good case when negotiating for a change of conditions or salary. The RCN and other trade unions have produced guidelines on the employment of practice nurses[20]. FHSA nurse advisers are usually very supportive. The following points should be considered in relation to employment.

Job description

A job description should specify the job title, the key activities and responsibilities, the clinical grade and salary, and to whom one is accountable. This can prevent misunderstanding if everyone involved knows what they are required to do. The RCN guidelines on clinical grading for practice nurses specify the type of work and the responsibility suitable to each grade[21].

Job descriptions also identify, by elimination, all the small tasks in a busy practice for which no-one has a definite responsibility. Unnecessary conflict can be prevented if such issues are resolved by discussion within the practice team.

Contract of employment

A contract of employment should cover: the salary and incremental dates, the hours of work, holiday entitlement, study leave, sick pay, maternity rights and benefits, pension arrangements (if any), and period of notice at the termination of the employment. In addition, the contract should set out the disciplinary and grievance procedures. If home visiting is part of the job description, then a mileage and car allowance should be negotiated[22].

Pensions

Pensions need careful consideration. Nurses coming into general practice from the NHS currently have to freeze their superannuation and start a private pension scheme, although this may change in the future. A few GPs contribute to staff pension funds, but most practice nurses have to make their own arrangements. Independent financial advice can be helpful in finding the most suitable scheme. A flexible plan which allows the contributions to be increased or decreased according to circumstances is often the best bet.

Insurance

National Insurance contributions, deducted at source from the salary, together with contributions made by the employer, pay for sickness and unemployment benefit and the state pension. GPs have indemnity insurance to cover vicarious liability for injury caused by their employees. However, personal indemnity insurance is essential because nurses as individuals can also be sued. The Royal College of Nursing and the Medical Defence Union provide indemnity insurance, and give legal advice to members if needed.

Accountability

Accountability for one's actions is one of the hallmarks of a professional person. Ultimately nurses are accountable to their patients, via the

UKCC, for the standards of nursing care provided. Among other things, the *Code of Professional Conduct* requires all nurses to refuse to accept delegated tasks for which they are not adequately trained[23]. Many aspects of practice nursing go far beyond what is taught pre-registration, and nurses may sometimes feel pressurised to take on work for which they are not adequately trained. The General Medical Council can discipline doctors for inappropriately delegating treatment or procedures[24], but nurses must be able to say 'no' when an activity is beyond their competence.

The *Scope of Professional Practice* outlines the criteria for developing the nursing role. It frees nurses from many of the previous petty restrictions, and allows them to accept new challenges; providing all the UKCC guidelines for safeguarding the public are followed[25].

Professional registration

Registration with the UKCC is required in order to practice as a nurse. The registration fee is paid three-yearly and each nurse is issued with a plastic card bearing a personal identification number (PIN). From April 1998 evidence of professional updating and learning will need to be available in a professional profile as part of the requirements for re-registration. A minimum of five study days in three years must be undertaken in subjects relevant to the area of work[26]. Many practice nurses already achieve much more than this[27], but arrangements are needed to help those who do not.

Networking for support

Practice nurses have traditionally been thought to work in greater isolation than other groups of nurses. This may be true in some instances; yet there is a large support network stretching out for those who look for it. Nurses who work in urban areas are likely to find contacts more easily than those in very remote areas, but the telephone and newsletters can be useful. Many practices now employ more than one practice nurse, so they can meet and support each other.

Local support

Most FHSAs employ a nurse adviser or facilitator. The facilitator posts began as a way of helping GPs to improve the prevention of coronary heart disease and strokes among their patients[28]. Nurse adviser posts came later as the FHSA members realised the need for a nursing input.

The development of all these posts has been varied. Some are still in their infancy, but where they have been most effective (for example in North East London), great strides have been made in practice nurse education. Money obtained from the Regional Health Authority has been used, among other things, to place contracts for practice nurse courses, family planning training, teaching and assessing, and nurse practitioner courses[29].

In some areas, practice nurse trainers are in post: experienced practice nurses with teaching qualifications, who act as community practice teachers (CPTs), similar to those for district nurses and health visitors. Training practices are also being designated, where a practice nurse has undertaken training in mentorship, or teaching and assessing, in order to provide support for students and newly qualified nurses.

Multidisciplinary training is being organised with some GPs, trainees, and other community nurses. However, in areas where there is no joint training in operation there is nothing to stop any nurse from contacting the local postgraduate medical centre, or community nursing head-quarters, and asking if joint meetings could be arranged.

Local practice nurse groups have developed spontaneously across the country. Groups of nurses meet to share ideas and hear speakers on topics of common interest. Nursing audit and quality control groups compare aspects of nursing practice and standards of care. A nurse who wished to start a group could contact all the general practices within a certain radius and invite the practice nurses to an inaugural meeting.

Some local groups keep a list of nurses available to take on locum cover. This would provide competent practice nurses who would be able to work in any practice setting at short notice.

Regional support

Many local practice nurse groups have affiliated to regional associations which have links with the RCN and Royal College of General Practitioners. Some regional associations provide grants for practice nurse education and research. The regional representatives can often work for change more effectively than individuals or small groups are able to do.

National support

The RCN Practice Nurse Association is very active on behalf of the members, and all the specialist groups within the RCN run study days and conferences. The Health Visitors' Association and District Nurses' Associations offer membership to practice nurses, and membership of Unison is open to all health service staff.

The National Practice Nurses Conference and Exhibition is planned and organised by a different regional group each year. About 500 nurses attend the three-day event, which provides a chance for social contact with colleagues as well as topical lectures and seminars.

Practice nurse education

The UKCC has decided its policy on community nurse education but the details still have to be worked out. Transitional arrangements are being made for experienced practice nurses to acquire the recordable qualification[30]. Newly qualified nurses will have a period of support from a nurse mentor, and nurses who have had a career break must undertake a back-to-nursing course before returning to practice. The wastage of the previous system, where any career move could mean complete retraining, is being replaced by a more integrated scheme. Two-thirds of the course for all community nurses will consist of subjects common to all the disciplines, followed by modules relevant to the eight different branches of community nursing. Enrolled nurses will be able to convert to first level nurses while undertaking the specialist nurse courses.

Many of these courses and modules involve distance learning and day release. Distance learning can be particularly suited to practice nurses, many of whom work part-time.

CATS, APEL and APL

Credit accumulation and transfer (CATS) is a way of evaluating the academic content of different courses so that points can be collected towards an academic award. Three levels of credit are awarded in England and Wales:

    120 credits at level 1 = certificate level
+ 120 credits at level 2 = diploma level
+ 120 credits at level 3 = degree level.

Scotland has four levels of credits (SCOTCATS)

Assessment of prior experiential learning (APEL) is a way of awarding credits for previous learning. Life experiences, professional knowledge and skills are assessed and credited towards a relevant academic course. A professional profile needs to be prepared, which outlines previous learning experiences and the ways they have influenced practice. Colleges usually charge for these assessments, which are complex to administer.

Assessment of prior learning allows credits to be awarded for relevant courses and examination results.

Identifying good practice

Audit

Audit means measuring what *is* being done, having made a prediction about what one *thinks* is being done. For example, a practice could have a policy for all diabetic patients to be reviewed annually, i.e. 100% of diabetic patients. Taking an audit would involve looking at the records of all patients with diabetes to see when they were last reviewed. As an example, it might turn out that only 85% of the patients were reviewed in the past year.

There is no point in doing this exercise unless the practice is prepared to act on the findings and take steps to remedy the deficiencies, but having done so, the audit should be repeated to see if the percentage rate has improved.

Local medical audit advisory groups (MAAGs) welcome nurse involvement in audit and will usually provide helpful advice and joint learning sessions. Nurses are also being employed by some organisations to advise on nursing audit.

Standards of care

Practice nurses have a particular need for ways of evaluating the quality of their work, because they so often work without supervision. The RCN Practice Nurse Association has produced a booklet on standards of care for practice nurses, as part of the wider Standards project[31].

Using this system, the components of each aspect of nursing work can be specified, and standard criteria written for each sub-topic. The standards to be met can be considered under the three headings devised by Donabedian[32].

- *Structure* – what resources are needed: facilities, equipment, personnel, education, record systems.
- *Process* – how the activity is carried out.
- *Outcome* – what effect the activity has on: the patient's health, knowledge or behaviour.

Specific standard statements can then be written, and each activity compared with the standard. Plans should then be formulated for improving any situation which falls below the ideal.

Other ways of monitoring quality can also be used. Peer review can be helpful if constructive criticism is offered. In such situations it helps if the person being reviewed first identifies what was good about the work, and then what could have been done better. The reviewer should then do the same[33]. Video recording is a useful way of assessing interactions with patients, but their written permission must be given before, and confirmed after, the consultation. Confidentiality must also be assured, and the tape cleared immediately after the review. Work is in progress in Lincolnshire on devising a quality audit tool for practice nurses[34].

District Health Authorities usually employ quality advisers who would be willing to advise practice nurses on assessing standards of care. In fact, most people with specialist knowledge are happy to share their expertise if they are asked.

Nursing research

Any new discipline has to establish itself by identifying and exploring the areas peculiar to it. Research explores these boundaries and establishes the body of knowledge required to practice the discipline. Research may be an academic and exhaustive study based in a university department, but it can be simply the questioning of routine procedures or asking the question 'why' in relation to day-to-day work. A practice nurse could be involved with research in several ways:

- keeping her/his own knowledge up-to-date – by reading research reports, or conducting a literature search on a particular topic,
- designing a study to test an idea for improving nursing practice,
- taking part in a wider research programme organised by a general practitioner, research nurse, or other outside body.

It is beyond the scope of this book to give detailed advice on research methodology but suggestions are given at the end of each chapter for possible ways of evaluating or investigating nursing practice. A few cardinal rules apply to research if worthwhile results are to be achieved:

- Identify the question to be answered and write it down. In formal research this is known as *stating a hypothesis*. In the example quoted above in *audit* the hypothesis would be that all patients with diabetes registered with the practice have an annual diabetic review.

- Conduct a *literature search* to find out what other people have done on this same subject. Librarians are usually very helpful if this seems daunting.
- Think how to go about answering the question and write it down. This is called the *protocol*. The *method* to be used may be a questionnaire, interviews or observation.
- Discuss the ideas, preferably with someone able to give impartial and constructive advice. Ensure that the research is *ethical*. Agreement will need to be obtained from the partners in the practice, especially if the study involves any of the patients. No patient should take part in research without giving his/her full consent.
- If a questionnaire is involved, get help designing it and then try it out on a few people to see if the questions are unambiguous and provide the answers being sought. Most questionnaires will need some revision after this *pilot survey*.
- Keep data collection simple and if in doubt refer back to the original question to see if it is *relevant* to that. The collection and statistical analysis of data is complex and in a large study would require expert help.
- If a *conclusion* is reached, make sure the result is *valid*. Was the size of the *sample* large enough? Could the results be due to chance alone? Were there too many *variables* to be able to attribute the results to one factor alone? Avoid making assumptions if they cannot be substantiated.
- Do something with the study after all that effort. This could mean organising a discussion with other members of the practice team about possible changes in policy, or writing a paper to give at a conference, or for publication in a journal.

Suggestions for evaluation and research

- Analyse your job description. Which elements constitute:
    - (a) treatment room work
    - (b) practice nurse work
    - (c) nurse practitioner work?

  Are there any activities which could be delegated?

  Are there any activities for which you need more training or supervision?
- What protection do you have against:
    - (a) wrongful dismissal?
    - (b) being sued for negligence?

- Review your professional profile. Does it provide a comprehensive picture of all your formal and experiential learning?
- Conduct a literature search on the ways of assessing the quality of nursing care in general practice.

References

1. News item (1993) Nurse sacked over smear test scandal; *Practice Nursing*, 21 September–4 October: 1
2. Lingard, P. (1994) GP's 'unorthodox technique prompts 300 smear recalls; *Pulse*, 19 March: 3.
3. Andrews, S. (1992) Sowing the seeds of practice nursing; *Practice Nurse*, **5:** 307–310.
4. Great Britain, Parliament (1968) *Health Services and Public Health Act*. HMSO, London.
5. Atkin, K., Lunt, N., Parker, G. and Hirst, M. (1993) *Nurses Count: a National Census of Practice Nurse*. Social Policy Research Unit, University of York.
6. DHSS (1986) *Neighbourhood Nursing – a Focus for Care*. HMSO, London.
7. Anon. (1986) The last word; *Journal of District Nursing*, **5** (4): 31.
8. Woolnough, F. (1990) A crisis of identity; *Practice Nurse*, **2:** 447–448, 454.
9. Audit Commission (1993) *Practice Makes Perfect: the Role of the Family Health Services Authorities*. HMSO, London.
10. Royal College of Nursing (1984) *The Training Needs of Practice Nurses – Report of the Steering Group*. RCN, London.
11. Walker, M. (1991) Is there a future for the community nurse practitioner? *Practice Nurse*, **4:** 11–16.
12. United Kingdom Central Council for Nurses, Midwives and Health Visitors (1986) *Project 2000: a New Preparation for Practice*. UKCC, London.
13. News (1994) PREP is passed but funding still unresolved; *Practice Nurse*, **7:** 255.
14. National Health Service Management Executive (1993) *Nursing in Primary Health Care: New Worlds – New Opportunities*. HMSO, London.
15. Jacka, S.M. and Griffiths, D.G. (1976) *Treatment Room Nursing: a Handbook for Nursing Sisters Working in General Practice*. Blackwell Scientific Publications, Oxford.
16. Bowling, A. and Stilwell, B. (Eds) (1988) *The Nurse in Family Practice*. Scutari Press, London.
17. Atkin, K., Lunt, N., Parker, G. and Hirst, M. (1993) *Nurses Count: a National Census of Practice Nurses*. SPRU, University of York.
18. Smith, M. (1993) Skill mix in general practice; *Practice Nursing*, 16 November–13 December: 21.
19. Ellis, N. (1994) *Employing Staff* (5th Edn). British Medical Journal, London.
20. UNISON (1993) *Conditions of Service for Practice Nurses – a Brief Guide*. UNISON, Regional Offices.

21. Royal College of Nursing (1993) *Guidance on the Employment of Nurses in General Practice.* RCN, London.
22. Royal College of Nursing (1993) *Guidance on the Employment of Nurses in General Practice:* 7. RCN, London.
23. UKCC (1992) *Code of Professional Conduct* (3rd Edn): para 4. UKCC, London.
24. General Medical Council (1993) *Professional Conduct and Discipline: Fitness to Practice:* para 42–3. GMC, London.
25. UKCC (1992) *The Scope of Professional Practice.* UKCC, London.
26. UKCC (1990) *The Report of the Post-Registration Education and Practice Project.* UKCC, London.
27. Atkin, K., Lunt, N., Parker, G. and Hirst, M. (1993) *Nurses Count: A National Census of Practice Nurses.* SPRU, University of York.
28. Astrop, P. (1988) Facilitator – the birth of a new profession; *Health Visitor,* **61** (19): 311–312.
29. News item (1992) Tailor-made training is a team effort; *Practice Nurse* **5:** 434–435.
30. United Kingdom Central Council for Nurses, Midwives and Health Visitors (1994) *The Future of Professional Practice – The council's standards for education and practice following registration.* UKCC, London.
31. Royal College of Nursing Standards of Care Project (1989) *A Framework for Quality.* Scutari, Harrow.
32. Donabedian, A. (1966) Evaluating the quality of medical care; *Milbank Memorial Fund Quarterly,* **44,** Part 2: 166–206.
33. Pendleton, D. *et al.* (1984) *The Consultation: An Approach to Learning and Teaching.* Oxford Medical Publications, Oxford.
34. Dutton, J. (1993) *Research into the Development of a Quality Audit Tool for Practice Nurses – Initial Survey.* North Lincolnshire Health Authority, Lincoln.

Further reading

Royal College of Nursing (1991) *Standards of Care for Practice Nursing.* Scutari, Harrow.
Wright, C. and Whittington, D. (Project co-ordinators) (1992) *Quality Assurance – an Introduction for Health Care Professionals.* Churchill Livingstone, Edinburgh.
Morton-Cooper, A. and Palmer, A. (1993) *Mentoring and Preceptorship – a Guide to Support Roles in Clinical Practice.* Blackwell Scientific Publications, Oxford.
Nolan, M. and Scott, G. (1993) Audit: an exploration of some tensions and paradoxical expectations; *Journal of Advanced Nursing,* **18:** 759–766.

Useful addresses

United Kingdom Central Council for Nurses, Midwives and Health Visitors.
23 Portland Place, London W1N 3AF
Telephone 071-637 7161

Royal College of Nursing
20 Cavendish Square, London W1M 0AB.
Telephone 071-409 3333.

Medical Defence Union
3 Devonshire Place, London W1N 2EA.
Telephone 071-486 6181.

Appendix 2.1
Examples of nursing journals

General nursing

Nursing Times
(Weekly): Macmillan Magazines

British Journal of Nursing
(Fortnightly): Mark Allen Publishing

Nursing Standard
(Weekly): Scutari Projects Ltd.

Journal of Advanced Nursing
(Monthly): Blackwell Scientific
Publications

Nursing (USA)
(Monthly): Springhouse Corp.

Journal of Clinical Nursing
(Bi-monthly): Blackwell Scientific
Publications

Professional Nurse
(Monthly): Mosby-Year Book Europe
Ltd.

Community nursing

Community Outlook
(Monthly): Macmillan Magazines
(free to community nurses)

Professional Care of Mother and Child
(Monthly): Media Medica
Publications Ltd
(free to community nurses)

*Health and Social Care in the
Community*
(Bi-monthly): Blackwell Scientific
Publications

Public Health Nursing (USA)
(Monthly): Blackwell Scientific
Publications Inc.

Primary Health Care
(Monthly): Scutari Projects Ltd
(free to community nurses)

General practice nursing

Practice Nurse
(20 issues per year): Reed Healthcare
Communications

Practice Nursing
(Fortnightly): Mark Allen Publishing
Ltd

Specialist subject journals

Healthlines
(10 issues per year): Health Education
Authority

*Journal of Psychiatric and Mental
Health Nursing*
(Bi-monthly): Blackwell Scientific
Publications

Journal of Wound Care
(10 issues per year): Macmillan
Magazines

Journal of Wound Care Nursing
Published by *Nursing Times* in
association with the Wound Care
Society.

Wound Management
(Bi-monthly): Media Medica
Publications
(free on request to nurses involved in
wound care)

Practical Diabetes
(Bi-monthly): PMH Medical
Publications
(free on request to named health
professionals involved with diabetes)

Diabetes Nursing
(Quarterly): Media Medica
Publications
(sponsored by Medisense)
(free on request to nurses involved in
diabetes care)

Asthma Practice
Colwood House Medical Publications
(Issued with *Practice Nurse*;
sponsored by Allen & Hanburys)

Chapter 3
Practice Organisation

Information about patients

The staff in general practice have access to a great deal of information, which raises important issues about the way that information is utilised and stored.

Confidentiality

Patients have a right to expect that any personal information about them will remain confidential. The ethical and confidential aspects of the work must be impressed on all staff members upon joining the practice, and the consequence of breaching confidentiality (instant dismissal) stated in the contract of employment.

The UKCC *Code of Professional Conduct* insists that nurses may only disclose confidential information: if the patient gives consent, if a court order is served, or if the wider public interest justifies the disclosure[1]. Naturally no nurse would deliberately flout this rule, but unwitting breaches can occur unless careful steps are taken to prevent them. There are risks to confidentiality in any of the following situations:

- conversations or telephone calls in the hearing of other patients,
- discussing a patient with a third party without consent,
- gossip about incidents which occur at work,
- records left lying open,
- information in the rubbish bin,
- computer screens which show other patients' details.

Computers with a 'screen-save' facility will go blank after a few minutes, but it is better to get into the habit of clearing the screen immediately after use.

Apart from heightened staff awareness, thought given to the design of reception and waiting areas and to sound-proofing consulting rooms can prevent conversations from being overheard. Manual records must be removed after use and filed as soon as possible and computer systems must be secure. If a shredding machine is not available, any waste paper which could identify patients must be torn up carefully or incinerated.

Investigation results should only be given to the person who had the test. This applies particularly to potentially sensitive investigations such as pregnancy tests. As a cautionary tale, picture the effect on the wife who was told her husband's post-vasectomy sperm count was negative, when she had already been sterilised!

There should be a practice policy to cover situations when a patient does not speak English. An interpreter should be arranged whenever possible, who is not a family member of the patient. In areas with mixed ethnic populations link workers are able to interpret and provide support[2].

Record system

A good record system is vital for the efficient management of patient care. The standard of records is expected to be high in vocational training practices, so that a GP trainee can have all the information about a patient available to him/her during a consultation.

Practice nurses are major contributors to the information system and to this end it is important to understand the records systems. The purpose of a record is:

- To record all the relevant information about a patient.
- To enable preventive care to be offered to appropriate patients.
- To facilitate the management of patients with chronic diseases.
- To enable all members of the PHCT to work together for the benefit of the patients.
- To act as a focus for the education of trainee GPs and other members of the PHCT.
- To enable data to be extracted for practice audit, performance review and research purposes.
- To provide evidence, if required, for medico-legal purposes.

The medical record envelope

The medical record envelopes, still known as 'Lloyd George envelopes' have been the main source of information about patients since they were introduced in 1911; the year that Lloyd George started a national health insurance scheme for working men[3]. The fact that the envelopes have been around so long says something for their durability, but also explains why in the 1990s their size may seem inadequate for today's needs. However, they are still in common usage and are capable of being adapted to meet most of the purposes outlined.

The continuation cards in the record should be in chronological order and tagged together. Letters should be trimmed to fit the envelope easily and all irrelevant material destroyed by the doctor. Letters and test results should also be tagged in chronological order.

Besides this simple and very basic record there are a number of insert cards which can be obtained to expand the information available.

Summary card

The summary card (contrarily pink for males and blue for females) is used to summarise all the important details about a patient. Inclusion of a summary card is a training requirement in many parts of the country, although much of this information is now held on computer instead.

Repeat prescription or treatment card

The various ways in which repeat prescriptions can be kept under control are more the responsibility of the office staff. However, an insert card with details of the present and recurrent treatment can be of value when a nurse is asked to obtain a repeat prescription for a patient. All requests must be entered on the card so that it is clear when the patient last had the item. A regular review by the doctor should be organised, because it is not desirable for any patient to have repeat prescriptions indefinitely.

Immunisation record cards

Immunisation record cards allow all the routine and travel vaccines given to be seen at glance. This makes it easier to see when immunisations have been missed, or reinforcing doses are due.

Contraceptive record card

Some practitioners use a contraceptive record card to ensure that routine items such as blood pressure check, cervical smear or contraceptive claim forms (FP1001/2) are not forgotten.

Screening

There are a number of other special record cards for health screening,

Over 75 checks, travel health or chronic disease management. The use of a range of other record cards is usually dictated by the enthusiasm of a practice for completing them and the size of the envelope in accommodating them.

A4 records

Mention has already been made of the small size of the 'Lloyd George' envelopes. Since the 1970s a number of practices have gone over to A4 (297 × 210 cm) records, the standard size for hospital notes. Fundholding generates a great deal of extra correspondence, which in turn causes storage problems. A4 records can then become inevitable, but they do take up more room.

Computers

Computerised record systems in general practice are now commonplace, and many doctors and nurses are enamoured with them. Their potential use is vast and the staff in computerised practices often wonder how they managed without one. Many practices still use manual records as well as computers, but the more adventurous ones are relying almost completely on their computers. The uses to which computers can be put is often limited by the training available. Regional user groups have been developed by the real enthusiasts, and it is worth at least one member of the practice joining. The information acquired can then be passed on to the rest of the staff. Apart from the obvious uses such as recording registration information, medical notes and details of preventive care, computers can be programmed for other purposes.

- *Prescriptions* can be printed. The computer will record all the relevant details, warn about possible drug interactions, and print a reminder when the patient needs a medication review.
- *Searches* can be made for a variety of reasons:
    - Call and recall of patients with specific medical conditions (e.g. asthma, diabetes, hypertension), or for preventive care (e.g. children for immunisation, women due for cervical smears, patients aged over 75).
    - Patients receiving a particular medication can be identified for research purposes, or audit (e.g. the number of prescriptions for influenza vaccine issued).
    - All the patients in a particular age range can be located (e.g. women age 40–50), or narrowed down further (e.g. women aged 50 who have had a hysterectomy and are not on HRT).

- *Word processing* can save time. Standard letters inviting patients for screening or immunisation can be saved in the computer and merged with the names and addresses of different patients to create personalised letters. Posters and information notices can be printed.

Links via the telephone lines through a modem will soon allow registration data to be sent directly to the FHSA, or pathology results to be received from the laboratory. However a modem also renders a computer system vulnerable to hackers who can invade a system for fun, or to access patient information. Entry to the system should be protected by codes and passwords which must be unique to each user and kept secret. Although computers are so exciting to use, there are other aspects to be considered as well. Under the terms of the Data Protection Act computer users have to be registered as data users[4]. This is usually arranged by the practice manager.

The machines are only as good as the people who write the programs and every system has some limitations. A fault in the program (bug) can lead to some bizarre results at times. A power failure or a fault with the equipment could cause essential patient information to be lost. For this reason daily copies of all the data must be made onto another disk or special tape, and a copy of this *back-up* kept off-site in case of fire or theft in the practice.

A plan of action should be prepared in case of a computer failure. All the users have a responsibility to protect the system as much a possible by following these simple rules:

- Do not write down any passwords. Protect them as safely as any cash card personal identification number.
- Keep the keyboards and terminals clean. No food or drinks should be allowed near a terminal.
- Exit from the system before switching off a terminal. Do not unplug any leads or move a terminal until it is switched off.
- Ask for help if anything unusual happens. DON'T PANIC.

The facilities and health protection required for staff who work with visual display units (VDUs) are laid down in the Health and Safety regulations[5].

Age/sex register

If a practice is not computerised a manual system for identifying patients will be needed. There are two types of manual register available: a book and a card file.

The book system

A looseleaf book may be used with each page representing a year (e.g. 1899, 1926 or 1978). All patients in the practice are recorded in the book under their year of birth and categorised by gender. Thus if all the patients born in 1980 were to be invited for tetanus and polio boosters, the page or pages relevant to that year could be consulted to find the patients' names.

The disadvantages of the book system are that only the patient's name can be recorded, and as patients leave the practice they are crossed out, so the pages soon look untidy.

The card system

The Royal College of General Practitioners has produced a set of pink and blue cards to organise an age/sex register. Each patient has an individual card which has space for other items of information to be recorded. The cards are then filed by year for males and females. This system is simple, inexpensive and effective.

Recall systems

Part of preventive care activities include recalling patients after a specified period of time. In the absence of a computer, a simple card system can be introduced along the lines of the age/sex register. Each patient has a card that is filed by the year and month when the patient is to be recalled. As each time interval comes up the patients concerned can be contacted by the practice secretary. A similar type of system can be used for many types of recall. Each card needs to be filed under the new date once the patient has attended. Patients who fail to attend will be easily spotted with this system.

Disease register

The age/sex cards can have coloured tags over the upper edge of the cards so that all the patients with a specific condition can be identified. Stickers can also be put on the patients' notes. The colour tagging system adopted by the RCGP became universally accepted. The code is:

Brown – diabetes
Yellow – epilepsy
Blue   – hypertension
Red   – sensitivity to drugs

Purple   –   cancer
Green   –   tuberculosis
Black   –   attempted suicide

This system gives the practice a modified disease register. Other colours and codes may be used which can prove to be confusing in the long run.

When first compiling a disease register, patients may be identified in several ways:

- at registration – during registration health checks,
- when diagnosed – if the GP diagnoses the condition, or a letter is received from a hospital,
- during consultations – when being seen for something else,
- from repeat prescriptions,
- from memory.

Once the patients' names are noted, their records can be checked to ensure there has been no mistake.

Computers are the easiest means of tracing patients with specific conditions, providing the diagnoses are entered in the first place. All systems ultimately rely on the conscientious input and updating of the data.

Access to records

In the past, medical records were jealously guarded from the eyes of the people most concerned – the patients themselves. As a result of which, sardonic comments in the notes, such as 'this patient enjoys very poor health', were not uncommon. Patients were not told the whole truth about their illness, especially if the prognosis was poor, and if the records later became mislaid a patient might never know what the original diagnosis had been.

The attitude to disclosure is now quite different and most patients expect to be given factual information. Patients have a legal right to see any information held about them in computer files[6]. A formal request in writing should be made. The doctor then has up to 40 days to provide the information, together with an explanation of any technical codes or abbreviations.

Since 1st November 1991 patients have also had a right of access to written records made after that date. The records of all health professionals, including nurses, are covered by the Access to Health Records Act (1990). A doctor can refuse to disclose information held manually or on computer:

- if he/she considers that serious mental or physical harm could be caused as a result, or
- to protect the confidentiality of a third party who might be identified from the patient's records[7].

If a request for access is received it can be helpful if a counselling interview is arranged to explore why the request was made. A patient may have unstated anxieties about his/her health, which could be allayed by a frank discussion. Alternatively, if there is dissatisfaction with any aspect of the treatment, the problem could be resolved amicably, in preference to a formal complaint to the FHSA. Where a policy of openness already exists, patients may have no need to resort to the law.

Nurses' own records

Many nurses write directly into the patients' NHS records. There can sometimes be a difference of opinion between doctors and nurses about such entries. Some doctors pride themselves on being able to write pithy one-liners, whereas nurses are taught to record a comprehensive, chronological account which covers:

- an assessment of the patients general health and the specific problems identified,
- the type of care planned,
- the nursing interventions made,
- the outcomes of the care given, and further actions planned or implemented[8].

In some instances, such as complicated wound care, or travel immunisation, separate nursing records can be more appropriate; especially where two or more part-time nurses are treating the same patient. Good communication is essential for continuity of care. Nursing records, if they are separate, should be amalgamated with the patients' notes when they are recalled by the FHSA.

Every nurse should have a copy of *Standards for Records and Record Keeping*, issued by the UKCC. This little booklet spells out clearly a nurse's responsibilities with regard to records. The data should be dated, written legibly in black ink, and signed by the person making the entry. Any alteration should be crossed through with a single line so it can still be read, and initialled[9]. The practice manager should keep a signature book, in case there is ever a query about a particular record.

Other records

A practice nurse may also choose to keep a *day-book* – a chronological account of all the interactions with patients. Any large book can be ruled up with columns for the information to be recorded. For example:

- Time seen – can be useful when auditing the workload or if a patient complains about having to wait.
- Name – to identify the patients seen. Date of birth can be included to make identification more specific.
- Contact – e.g. S (surgery), V (visit) or T (telephone).
- Activity – a brief note or abbreviation of the reason for the consultation.
- Comments – can be an *aide-memoire* for further action e.g. 'notes' (if not available at the time of the consultation), 'FP73' (if a claim form has to be written).
- Initials – the nurse who saw the patient (if more than one nurse on duty).

A day-book can be useful for auditing nursing activities and for checking back if there are any queries about a patient's visit. With a suitable computer system much of this information can be entered and retrieved that way, in which case a day-book becomes irrelevant.

Private patients

Many practices are now Yellow Fever Centres providing immunisation for patients who are not registered with the practice. There is no official record for private patients, (unlike those for registered patients and temporary residents), but if injections are given privately, then a system must be devised for recording information about each patient and the immunisation given (see Chapter 5, *Injections*).

Policies and protocols

When a nurse joins a practice she/he will need to discuss the nursing role with the doctors. The exact scope and responsibility of each nurse will be governed by her/his previous experience and training. The limits of a nurse's freedom to act autonomously should be negotiated, and then recorded in a *protocol*. This word is used rather freely and can be viewed as either a protection or a threat. If a protocol is too rigid then any deviation from it could place a practitioner at risk of prosecution, should anything go wrong. This is a particular concern of doctors, who fear being constrained to provide medical treatment exactly as specified in a treatment protocol[10].

On the other hand, many nurses feel they can work with greater confidence if they have agreed boundaries. Protocols should make clear the nurse's role and responsibilities for particular activities and when a referral should be made to the general practitioner. The RCN has produced a book of guidelines for writing protocols[11], but every practice will need to agree their own because so much depends on the individual nurse's experience and competence.

Policies

Policies or rules are needed in any organisation so that all the staff know what is expected of them. Some policies in general practice are dictated by legal statute or public safety requirements. For example:

- Health and safety issues in accordance with the Health and Safety at Work directives[12].
- Fire regulations – covering the maintenance of fire extinguishers, staff training, and the procedure in the event of a fire.
- Control of infection – covering the handling of specimens, dealing with body fluids, the disposal of sharps and clinical waste, methods of preventing cross-infection.

Other policies may cover more domestic issues such as: the arrangement of holidays and study leave, setting healthy examples for the public, avoiding waste of energy and resources.

Meetings

Clinical meetings between members of the primary health care team are essential for exchanging information and giving feedback about patients, as well as providing learning opportunities for all concerned. Support can also be offered to individual team members who are dealing with stressful situations.

Joint staff meetings are valuable when domestic policies are being decided. Compliance will be better if everyone has been consulted and understands the need for the policy. 'Off the cuff' pronouncements, which are subsequently changed, can be very damaging for morale. Team meetings need to be structured so that everyone is able to make a valid contribution, and when decisions are reached, everyone likely to be affected must be made aware of them.

Social gatherings, like a Christmas party or summer barbeque, can cement good relationships within the team. The more that people meet together informally and formally, the better they will know each other and understand each other's role.

Appointments

Practices have different ways of arranging access for patients to the GP or practice nurse. With a simple queuing system patients arrive at the beginning of surgery and are seen on a first-come, first-served basis. If a number is given to each patient on arrival they can be called in turn without the fear of jumping the queue or being missed out. Single-handed practices often operate a queuing system successfully, but they also tend to offer less of the extra services provided by group practices[13].

Appointment systems allow the workload to be spaced out and planned in advance, which in theory should save patients from having to wait more than a few minutes to be seen. However patients cannot be ill by appointment, so time must always be set aside for dealing with urgent problems. If an emergency arises during surgery time, the booked appointments are likely to be delayed. Most people will accept such delays providing they are kept informed and do not feel they are being treated unfairly.

Computerised appointment systems are now more common. These can log the time a patient arrived, when the patient was seen, and even how long the consultation took – all valuable information for auditing the effectiveness of the organisation. Even without a computer, audits can be conducted to identify ways of improving the system.

If patients do not keep their appointments, this is not only a waste of professional time, it can also deprive other patients of the chance to be seen sooner. A graph in the waiting area, showing the number of hours wasted by non-attenders each week, can be helpful in educating the public about their responsibilities towards the service. Some practices and health centres run consumer groups where patient representatives can make suggestions for improving the organisation.

Practice nurses who use appointment systems can give the receptionists a list of the time to be allowed for specific procedures and consultations. Blood tests may need to be done in the morning before the courier calls to collect them, while counselling and health promotion are better suited to quieter times. Some activities such as travel health, diabetes or asthma care, may be undertaken in specific clinics. Alternatively, a policy of allowing patients to select times to suit themselves may increase the number of people who are able to attend for health promotion and screening.

Investigation results

A system is needed for ensuring that patients get the results of investigations. A patient must either know when to return to see the doctor, or when to telephone for results. Abnormal results should not be filed until the necessary steps have been taken for the patient to be followed up.

Telephone calls

A policy is needed for the handling of telephone calls. Too many interruptions during surgery time can be disruptive, but patients have to be put through in urgent situations. Other callers can be given a time to call back; although no patient should have to ring more than twice. Some doctors and nurses overcome this problem by having allotted telephone times for giving test results, or dealing with other enquiries. Any advice given over the telephone should be recorded in the patient's records, and telephone messages should be written down immediately in case they get forgotten.

Organisation is a complex but essential area of general practice. The fundamental message is that all members of the team should feel involved in the success of the practice. Good ideas can be disseminated through regular team visits to other practices.

Suggestions for evaluation and research

- Sit in the waiting area for 10–15 minutes and note any information you hear about any of the patients.
- Audit a random sample of patient records in which nursing activities are recorded. How many records meet the standards specified by the UKCC for record-keeping?
- Conduct a literature search on the value of protocols.
- Devise an anonymous questionnaire to discover the patients' satisfaction with the practice arrangements for access to the practice nurse(s).

References

1. United Kingdom Central Council for Nurses, Midwives and Health Visitors (1992) *Code of Professional Conduct* (3rd Edn), paragraph 10. UKCC, London.
2. Bowler, H. (1993) Seeing health in black and white (using advocates); *Practice Nurse*, **6:** 622.

3. Alsopp, J. (1984) *Health Policy and the National Health Service:* 22. Longman, London.
4. Great Britain, Parliament (1984) *The Data Protection Act 1984.* HMSO, London.
5. Health and Safety Executive (1992) *Display Screen Equipment Work – Guidance on Regulations Health and Safety (Display Screen Equipment) Regulations (1992).* HMSO, London.
6. Panting, G. (1990) *The Data Protection Act 1984; Update,* **41**(2): 127–129.
7. Dimond, B. (1991) A question of access; *Nursing Standard,* **6**(4): 18–19.
8. Marriner, A. (1979) *The Nursing Process – a Scientific Approach to Nursing Care* (2nd Edn). Mosby, USA.
9. UKCC (1993) *Standards for Records and Record Keeping.* UKCC, London.
10. Pitts, J.R. (1993) Protocols for acute conditions; *Update,* **47** (12): 785–786.
11. Smail, J. *Protocols for Health Promotion Clinics.* RCN and South Glamorgan FHSA.
12. Health and Safety Commission (1992) *Workplace Health, Safety and Welfare – Approved Code of Practice (Health, Safety and Welfare) Regulations 1992.* HMSO, London.
13. Food and Health (1993) GP Access, *Which,* March: 11–14.

Further reading

McGee, P. (1992) *Teaching Transcultural Care.* Chapman & Hall, London.
Elliott-Binns, C., Bingham, L. and Peile, E. (Eds) (1992) *Managing Stress in the Primary Health Care Team.* Blackwell Scientific Publications, Oxford.

Useful addresses

Health and Safety Executive Information Centre
Broad Lane, Sheffield S3 7HQ.
Telephone 0742-822344. *Fax* 0742-892333.

Chapter 4
Management of the Nurses' Rooms

As the work in general practice and the number of nurses expands or contracts, the accommodation needed by the practice nurses can change. The basic requirements include:

- a treatment/consulting room with access to a toilet for the patients,
- a room for use as a recovery room,
- a waiting area for patients,
- a secure store-room,
- a safe area for storing clinical waste and sharps before collection,
- access to a changing room, and refreshment area or common room.

The practice nurse(s) should be involved when new or extended buildings are planned. The extra rooms, or refinements to the nurses' accommodation might then include:

- a separate consulting room,
- an annexe to the treatment room for dealing with used instruments and specimens etc., and an adjacent toilet with a hatch for patients' specimens,
- an office space for administration,
- a separate minor surgery room,
- access to a non-clinical room for counselling,
- room for group sessions,
- facilities for mothers and babies.

There are recommendations on premises: on ease of access, toilet facilities for wheelchair users, size of waiting areas etc. in the 'Red Book'. It stipulates that treatment rooms should be at least 17.5 square metres[1]. In addition, there are Health and Safety requirements on heating, ventilation, lighting and other aspects of the workplace[2].

Design and furnishing

Even in less than ideal premises a better environment can be created by the imaginative use of space and colour. A filing cabinet and bright, stackable, plastic crates can reduce clutter. Leaflet racks on the walls make information easily accessible, and pinboards are better than adhesive tape for displaying travel charts and other reference material.

Attractive decor will create a welcoming atmosphere. Light, cool colours give a feeling of space; and warm tones, a more friendly effect. Many people are nervous in a clinical environment; pictures, plants, and toys for children can help put them at ease. Well-kept notice boards dealing with seasonal topics have more impact than walls smothered with depressing posters condemning every human weakness.

Lighting should be chosen with care. Bright even lighting is needed in treatment areas. Warm-tone fluorescent tubes are less cruel. Directable lamps are needed for minor surgery, cervical smears and ear syringing. Softer lighting from lamps or wall-lights is desirable for counselling or teaching relaxation. Blinds can control the entry of bright sunlight, and be used to give privacy when needed.

Basic furnishings include a desk, chairs, couch, lockable cupboards, and bookshelves. A curtained area or screen gives extra privacy for the patients, and a mirror is helpful when they are getting dressed. A box of washable toys for children is essential.

Treatment and minor surgery couches should be accessible from all sides, and be height-adjustable for ease of working[3]. A secure step is needed for patients to get onto a non-adjustable couch.

Patients will feel less intimidated if sitting at the same level as the nurse at the side of the desk, not being confronted across it. Low chairs away from the desk are preferable for counselling and informal discussions. Furniture should be arranged so that the nurse's exit is not obstructed if a patient becomes aggressive (see Chapter 14). An alarm bell is needed for summoning help in any sort of emergency.

Work surfaces and flooring in treatment areas should be hard-wearing, easy to clean and able to withstand bleach (in case of blood-spillage). Sinks should have elbow taps and minimise splashing to prevent cross-infection. A separate sink should be available for washing used instruments, and a 'dirty' work area designated, for dealing with specimens etc.

All emergency equipment must be easily accessible. A visible plan of the storage areas can save a nurse from returning to a scene of devastation after a day off!

Health and safety

Although work areas are planned for practicability, the overwhelming consideration should be for the safety of the public and staff. Employers are legally required to produce a safety policy[4] and to report serious incidents to the Health and Safety Executive (HSE)[5]. All employees have a duty to take reasonable care to avoid injury to themselves or others and to co-operate with employers in meeting the statutory requirements of the Health and Safety at Work Act[6]. The area officers of the Employment Medical Advisory Service (EMAS), part of the HSE, will give advice and provide literature on all aspects of occupational health[7].

Control of substances hazardous to health (COSSH)

Employers are required to carry out a risk assessment for any substance which could be hazardous to health[8]. The assessment should cover:

- the name of the substance,
- the type of hazard and precautions to be taken,
- the planned use of the substance,
- possible unplanned events and the action to be taken.

Any staff member likely to be exposed to substances hazardous to health must understand the risks and the precautions to be taken. Hazardous substances which might be used in general practice include:

Ethyl chloride	Phenol
Formaldehyde	Potassium permanganate
Glutaraldehyde	Silver nitrate
Industrial spirit	Sodium hypochlorite solution
Contaminated waste	

Special precautions are needed if a mercury sphygmomanometer is broken, because the fumes can be toxic. The mercury should be contained within the apparatus if possible, or be tipped into an airtight container, covered with water, and sealed. Mercury spillage kits are available, with special absorbent sponges, and containers for storing the mercury for disposal. Detector pads left in the vicinity of the spillage will change colour if mercury fumes are present. The kits can be purchased, or a local pharmacist might be willing to provide an emergency service, for a fee.

Supplies and equipment

The amount of clinical equipment needed varies from practice to practice (see Appendix 4.1). The practice nurse is responsible for ensuring the proper upkeep, and for knowing the correct way to use the equipment in her/his care. Instruction booklets and guarantees should be kept on file. Any faulty equipment must be withdrawn from use, labelled, and reported to the practice manager or general practitioner. Maintenance contracts are needed for essential, or potentially dangerous items such as autoclaves.

Ordering supplies and equipment

Practice policy will determine who has the responsibility for ordering supplies. Whether nurses place orders directly, or via the practice manager, everyone has a responsibility for seeking value for money. Discounts may be available for bulk orders, but it is false economy if the items do not have a long enough shelf-life. Be warned – some items may appear cheaper by mail order, but can attract very expensive delivery charges. Some sources of supply:

Source	Product examples
Direct purchase from manufacturer.	Travel and other vaccines, nebuliser spares.
Purchase from wholesaler or medical mail order firm.	Examination equipment, instruments, gloves, paper couch rolls, diaphragms.
Purchase on account from local pharmacy.	Dressings, drugs, lotions.
On prescription from local pharmacy.	Replacement of items used in emergency – dressings and injections for named patients.
Requisition from FHSA.	Syringes, needles, NHS stationery.
Requisition from District Hospital. Or: Requisition from the vaccine distributor.	Pathology forms, specimen containers, childhood vaccines.
Requisition from Health Promotion Department.	HP leaflets/posters, loan of resources, videos etc.
Contract with FHSA, local authority or private contractor.	Collection of clinical waste and sharps. Supply sharps bins and yellow bags.

Purchase from cash and carry.   Cleaning materials, batteries, pillows,
                                        paper towels.

Copies of requisitions and receipts need to be kept for audit and accounting purposes.

Emergency equipment

Every practice must have a basic supply of emergency drugs and equipment, which is easily accessible. The exact items to be kept should be agreed with the doctor. The practice nurse is usually responsible for checking and maintaining the level of emergency supplies. Adrenaline has a short shelf-life and will need to be replaced regularly. All items must be purchased initially but any drugs used can then be replaced on prescription. (See Appendix 4.2 *Emergency equipment*).

Training in emergency procedures

As many staff as possible should be able to undertake basic life-support measures in emergencies. People tend to go to the surgery in time of trouble but there may not always be a doctor or nurse in the building. The practice nurse might help to organise first-aid training for other staff. Resuscitation training can usually be arranged through the district resuscitation training officer.

Fire precautions

Every practice should have a procedure for dealing with a fire, and an adequate supply of appropriate fire extinguishers. These need to be serviced at least annually and staff trained in their use.

The storage of medicines and other substances

Controlled drugs are regulated under the Misuse of Drugs Act (1971). They must be stored in a special locked cupboard which is out of sight of windows and the public. A register must be kept on the premises for recording any new stock, the date it was obtained and the dispensing of any of the stock to patients, or to individual doctors for their emergency bags. Out-of-date or unwanted controlled drugs may only be destroyed by persons authorised under the Act[9].

The Misuse of Drugs Act was the successor to the original Dangerous Drugs Act, and was intended to provide a more flexible and comprehensive control over the misuse of drugs of all kinds. The drugs covered are divided into three categories, according to the harmfulness of the drug when it is misused e.g.:

● Class A – cocaine, diamorphine, dipipanone, methadone, morphine and pethadine.
● Class B – oral amphetamines, cannabis, codeine and pholcodeine.
● Class C – certain drugs related to the amphetamines.

Care must be taken with all drugs, lotions and cleaning materials. They should always be kept in locked cupboards; but because on occasions in a busy treatment room a cupboard might be left unlocked, extra precautions are also sensible:

● All liquids should have child-proof bottle tops and be stored out of reach of children. (The unfortunate child who gained access to a consulting room and drank some phenol proved the need for such precautions[10].)
● Quick-release safety catches on cupboard doors and fridges will help to deter inquisitive toddlers.
● Clear all trolleys after use. (Imagine the effect of a silver nitrate pencil used as a play lipstick.)

Storage of vaccines

A doctor or nurse could be prosecuted for negligence for vaccination failure as a result of inadequate storage if it could be shown that the cold chain was intact before the product reached the practice[11]. Vaccines must be stored at the temperatures specified by the manufacturers. This is no easy task since oral polio vaccine requires a temperature range of 0 to 4°C while most other vaccines need to be between 2 and 8°C. It does not take a mathematician to realise the narrow range between 2 and 4°C is all they have in common. Special vaccine fridges have a thermostatically controlled temperature range between 2 and 6°C.

Maximum/minimum thermometers are essential for continuous temperature monitoring in all refrigerators. A digital thermometer with a probe attached to a flexible wire can be used to 'map' the temperature variations within the refrigerator. That way, the polio vaccine can be stored in the coolest area. The display part of the digital thermometer can be fixed to the wall outside the fridge, so that the temperature can be seen at all times. The flexible wire passing into the fridge will not affect the door closure.

If the cold chain is broken the vaccine may have to be destroyed. Seek advice from a pharmacist, or the vaccine manufacturers, in such an event.

Recommendations for vaccine storage

Action	Rationale
A named person to be responsible for vaccines.	To ensure that the regulations are followed
Check and record min./max. temperatures daily.	To ensure that the correct temperature has been maintained throughout the 24 hours, and as proof of regular monitoring.
Defrost refrigerator regularly.	For most efficient and cost-effective running.
Store vaccines in a cold-box or another fridge while defrosting.	To maintain the cold-chain.
Have the refrigerator wired in, or keep a dedicated socket for it.	So it cannot be turned off inadvertently.
Make sure the fridge door closes properly.	To maintain the correct temperature at all times.
Do not load more than 50% of the fridge, and allow room between the batches of vaccines on each shelf.	Temperatures are maintained more easily if the air can circulate freely[12].
Do not over-order vaccines.	To ensure they are not kept too long, or pass their expiry date.
Do not store food etc., in a vaccine fridge.	To reduce the need to open the door unnecessarily, and to comply with Health and Safety Regulations[13].

Control of infection

Measures to prevent the spread of infection are needed in general practice. People who might be infectious should be tactfully taken to a waiting room away from other patients, and staff members who are ill ought to stay at home when necessary. There should be a practice *Control of Infection* policy and appropriate training provided. The RCN has produced guidelines for practice nurses[14].

Hand washing

Elbow taps, soap dispensers and paper towels are needed in the toilets and clinical areas to reduce hand-to-hand contamination. Bacteria have been shown to multiply on moist bar soap and reusable towels[15]. Alcohol and chlorhexidine (*Hibisol*) can be used as an alternative to hand washing if necessary. Hand disinfectant solutions (e.g. *Hibiscrub*) should be used prior to invasive procedures[16].

Protective clothing

The 'great uniform debate' seems to have less to do with protection than with image. Some nurses prefer to maintain a traditional image, while others choose to be less formal. In a recent study, the patients interviewed liked a female nurse who performs tasks and procedures to wear a uniform dress; but they preferred a smart skirt and blouse for a nurse who gives counselling and advice[17].

Whatever is worn, disposable aprons should be used for procedures likely to contaminate clothing. Gloves are needed when there is any risk of transmitting or contracting any infection. Sterile surgeons' gloves must be used for invasive procedures: minor surgery or inserting IUDs and for dressing major wounds such as burns. Unsterile latex gloves are adequate for phlebotomy, minor dressings, and performing rectal or vaginal examinations.

Masks and eye protection should be available if there is any risk of blood being splashed into the mouth or eyes. Such risks are uncommon in general practice, but if a risk is present then facilities for eye irrigation are also needed[18].

All the staff need to be familiar with the procedure for dealing with body fluids when accidents occur. Although HIV infection causes the most concern, the virus is less easily transmitted than hepatitis B. Much smaller amounts of hepatitis B virus are needed, and it is stable in organic matter outside the body for long periods.

Hepatitis B infection

The virus is spread by contact with infected body fluids through inoculation, or contact with broken skin and mucous membranes. Any cuts or breaks in the skin should be covered with waterproof plaster.

General practitioners and practice nurses need to be immunised against hepatitis B, and have their immunity checked. A record should be kept of the immunisation dates and checks of antibody levels. There should also be a practice policy on needle-stick injuries.

Human immunodeficiency virus (HIV) infection

Three factors must apply before HIV can be transmitted:

- *Amount* – there must be enough of the virus. HIV can be found in high concentrations in blood, semen and vaginal secretions of infected people. Sweat, tears, saliva, urine and faeces contain much less concentrated amounts[19].
- *Condition* – HIV deteriorates rapidly outside the body and is destroyed by heat, bleach and detergents. The enzymes in saliva and gastric acid also attack the virus.
- *Route of infection* – there must be a way into the bloodstream.

The most common means of spread are by unprotected sexual intercourse, sharing unclean equipment for I/V drug use, or from mother to child. Infected blood inside a used needle could be injected during a needle-stick injury. HIV has on rare occasions been contracted by individuals with severe eczema. The macrophages in the exudate of the eczematous lesions are thought to have ingested the virus in infected blood in contact with the skin[20].

Practice nurses have a role in educating people about HIV infection. That means separating the myths from the facts and having up-to-date knowledge. HIV/AIDS awareness days are regularly run by district health, and local authorities. HIV/AIDS specialist nurses will provide guidance if asked.

Needle-stick injuries

A strict adherence to the procedure for the use of sharps will prevent all but the most untoward accidents. If a needle-stick injury occurs the following action should be taken immediately:

Action	Rationale
Encourage the puncture wound to bleed freely. Wash the area under running water.	To flush any organisms from wound.
Irrigate with plenty of water any mucous membranes exposed.	Micro-organisms can gain entry through aerosols of blood in contact with mucous membranes.
Report the injury to the employing GP.	An accident report will have to be made out and tests may be needed.

Ask the patient to wait (if known).

Blood tests may be requested. Tests can be performed with consent, for Hep.B antigen, but counselling is necessary before testing for HIV antibodies.

Blood tests may be taken from the person injured.

As a baseline against later tests for Hep.B and HIV.

Immunisation against hepatitis B may be needed (if not immune).

(See Chapter 11)

Disinfection and sterilisation

Every practice should have a policy for the decontamination of equipment. Central sterile supply (CSSD) is the ideal way of ensuring a regular standard of sterile equipment, but the service may be unavailable or too costly for many practices. Single-use disposable items should be used whenever possible. The practice nurse is usually responsible for decontaminating non-disposable surgical and examination equipment. A thorough understanding of the principles is needed. Equipment may be treated according to the level of risk:

- *Low risk* – aural specula, ear syringe nozzles (used for non-infected ears).
- *Moderate risk* – vaginal specula, practice diaphragms, aural specula and syringe nozzles (used for infected ears), nebulisers.
- *High risk* – minor surgery instruments, speculum and instruments for inserting IUDs[21].

Cleansing

All washable equipment must be thoroughly cleaned with hot water and detergent, and rinsed thoroughly. Household gloves should be worn, and splashing avoided. Blood or debris dried on the surface of an instrument will prevent adequate sterilisation. Pre-soaking may be necessary. Brushes used for cleaning equipment must be autoclaved and replaced regularly, and stored dry. A *cytobrush* (for cervical smears) is the ideal size for cleaning aural specula.

Sterilisation

Sterilisation destroys micro-organisms and spores and is the only safe method of decontamination for 'high-risk' instruments. Autoclaving is the most effective method of sterilisation in general practice[22].

Autoclaves

This process uses steam under pressure to sterilise instruments and other equipment. Autoclaves can be obtained in different sizes, but they are required to meet British Standard specifications[23]. Sterilisation may be achieved with high temperatures for a short period, or with longer cycles at lower temperatures. In order to be effective the appropriate temperature must be maintained for the correct length of time (Fig. 4.1). The time taken to reach a temperature and to cool down afterwards is immaterial. The highest temperature can be used for metal instruments, and the lowest for plastics and practice diaphragms if used.

The reservoir must be filled with distilled water, and the water level checked regularly. Thrice yearly servicing is recommended, and emergency repairs as necessary. The full cycle should be observed regularly to check the temperatures and timing. Newer autoclaves, such as the SES 2000 can provide a printout of the sterilisation data.

The steam must be able to reach all the surfaces of an object. The blades of instruments must be open, and overloading of the trays

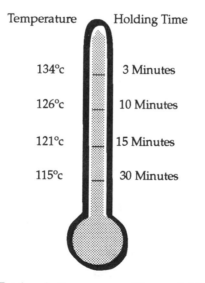

Temperature		Holding Time
134°c		3 Minutes
126°c		10 Minutes
121°c		15 Minutes
115°c		30 Minutes

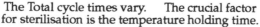

The Total cycle times vary.   The crucial factor
for sterilisation is the temperature holding time.

Fig. 4.1 Autoclave sterilisation.

avoided. Gallipots and receivers should be placed on their sides. Instruments can be sterilised in pouches in autoclaves which have a drying cycle. Special racks are needed to keep the pouches separate and in a vertical position.

A practice policy is needed to ensure contaminated equipment is never put into the autoclave until ready to start the sterilisation process. That way, unsterile equipment cannot be taken out of the autoclave and reused by mistake.

Hot air ovens

Instruments can be sterilised by dry heat in hot air ovens, but higher temperatures are needed for longer periods than for autoclaving (Fig. 4.2). Ideally the oven should be fan-assisted to ensure an even temperature distribution.

Chaetles forceps should be kept in a clean, dry holder next to the autoclave or oven, and be used only for removing sterile objects. The forceps should be autoclaved daily and the holder washed and dried well.

Disinfection

Chemical disinfectants and boiling water can destroy bacteria and other micro-organisms but do not destroy spores.

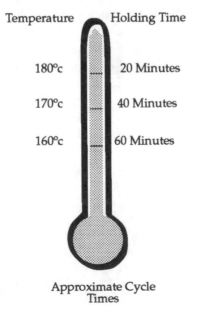

Temperature		Holding Time
180°c		20 Minutes
170°c		40 Minutes
160°c		60 Minutes

Approximate Cycle
Times

Fig. 4.2　Hot air sterilisation.

Hot water disinfectors

Clean instruments can be immersed in water and boiled vigorously for at least five minutes after the water starts boiling again. The disinfector should not be overloaded, and the process must be timed accurately. The water should be changed regularly.

Chemical disinfection

Chemicals may be used for 'low and medium risk' items like thermometers, and items which cannot be autoclaved, such as nebuliser chambers and masks. Endoscopes, if they are used in general practice, can be disinfected with glutaraldehyde, but special precautions are needed to comply with the COSSH regulations because glutaraldehyde produces toxic fumes. Alcohol and hypochlorites are most commonly used in general practice.

Industrial methylated spirit can be used to disinfect clean, heat-sensitive items. Ten minutes immersion time is needed.

Sodium hypochlorite, as household bleach and *Milton*, can be used in dilution for 30 minutes to disinfect plastics and glass. The dilutions needed depend on the brand. The instructions on the label should be followed. Nebuliser chambers and masks, aural specula and nozzles for pulsed water units, injection trays, spoons used for polio drops, and bowls used to wash feet, are suitable for this treatment.

Sodium dichloroisocyanurate (NaDCC) tablets can be dissolved in water to give a more reliable dilution of chlorine. NaDCC granules (*Presept*) can be used to disinfect blood and other body fluids. All the staff should be aware of the procedure if a spillage occurs:

Action	Rationale
Put on household gloves.	To avoid hand contact.
Cover the spillage with chlorine granules or a 1% hypochlorite solution. Leave for ten minutes.	To inactivate any micro-organisms.
Remove any broken glass with forceps.	To avoid accidental cuts.
Cover the spillage with paper towels, scoop it up and place in a yellow bag.	To be incinerated as clinical waste.

Use hot water and strong detergent for surfaces, such as carpets, which cannot tolerate bleach.

The disposal of clinical waste

The Environment Protection Act (1990) requires everybody who produces clinical waste to ensure that:

- The waste is stored correctly until collected.
- A written description of the waste is supplied.
- The waste is transferred to a registered carrier[24].

Blades, needles and syringes must be deposited in sharps containers which meet the British Standard BS 7320:1990. The containers must be kept out of reach of children. A child recently sustained a needle-stick injury in a general practice, through reaching into a used sharps bin[25].

Dressings and other soft waste contaminated with blood or body fluids must go into yellow bags. The sharps bins and yellow bags must be stored in a locked room or cupboard inaccessible to the public. The waste must be able to be traced back to the person responsible. Unwanted medicines must also be disposed of safely to comply with the terms of Environment Protection Act. A GP was prosecuted and found to be negligent after the drugs given to a pharmacist for disposal were dumped[26].

The practice must have a contract for a regular collection of the clinical waste. On no account must it be put into the ordinary rubbish bins.

Suggestions for evaluation and research

- Organise with the practice manager an emergency procedure practice. Assess the results:
    - (a)   Did everyone know what to do?
    - (b)   Was all the emergency equipment available?
    - (c)   Could anything have been done better?
- Review all the storage and disposal facilities in the nurses' rooms. Do they meet all the legal requirements?
- Review:
    - (a)   The facilities for counselling patients in the nurses' rooms.
    - (b)   The procedures for decontaminating equipment in your practice.

Prepare a report, including appropriate references, if any changes are needed.

References

1. Department of Health, Welsh Office (1990) Notes on standards of practice accommodation; *Statement of Fees and Allowances to General Medical Practitioners in England and Wales from April 1990*: para 56, schedule 1. NHS General Medical Services.
2. HSC (1992) Workplace Health, Safety and Welfare – Approved Code of Practice – Workplace (Health, Safety and Welfare) Regulations 1992. HMSO, London.
3. HSE leaflet *Ergonomics at Work IND* (9) 9OL 5OM 5/90.
4. HSC booklet, *Writing a Safety Policy Statement: Advice to Employers*. HSC 6 C1000 8/91.
5. HSE booklet *The Reporting of Injuries or Dangerous Occurrences Regulations 1985*. HSE 11(Rev) 100M 9/90.
6. HSE (1992) *Essentials of Health and Safety at Work* (Rev. Edn). HMSO, London.
7. HSE leaflet (1992) *An Introduction to the Employment Medical Service*. HSE 5 8/92 250C.
8. *Control of Substances Hazardous to Health Regulations* (1988), made under the *Health and Safety at Work Act 1974*. HMSO, London.
9. Department of Health (1989) *Guide to the Misuse of Drugs Act 1971 and the Misuse of Drugs Regulations*. HMSO, London.
10. News item (1992) Doctor faces charge after child drank acid; *Daily Telegraph*, 19 September.
11. Haworth, E., Booy, R., Stirzaker, L., Wilkes, S. and Battersby, A. (1993) Is the cold chain for vaccines maintained in general practice? *British Medical Journal* **307**: 242–4.
12. Grassby, P. (1992) *Safe Storage of Vaccines: Problems and Solutions*. St Mary's Hospital, Penarth, S. Glamorgan.
13. Kerr, V. (1993) Cool the hot topic of vaccine storage; *Practice Nurse*, **6**: 732, 736.
14. Royal College of Nursing (1994) *Guidelines on Infection Control for Nurses in General Practice*. RCN, London.
15. Mendes, M. and Lynch, D. (1976) A bacteriological survey of wash-rooms and toilets; *Journal of Hygiene*, Cambs. **76**: 183–190.
16. Reybrook, G. (1986) Handwashing and hand disinfection; *Journal of Hospital Infection*, **8**: 5–23.
17. Rowland, W. (1994) Patients' perceptions of nurse uniforms; *Nursing Standard*, **8** (19): 32–36.
18. British Medical Association (1989) *A Code of Practice for Sterilisation of Instruments and Control of Cross-Infection*. BMA, London.
19. Notman, A. and Mackenzie, A. (1993) Handling HIV; *Nursing Times*, **89** (26): 34–35.
20. See no. 19.

21. Hoffman, P., Cooke, E.M., Larkin, D.P., Southgate, L.J., Mayon White, R.T., Pether, J.V.S. and Wright, A.E. (1988) Control of infection in general practice; *British Medical Journal*, **297:** 34–36.
22. News (1993) Sterilise with steam, not hot air; *Practice Nurse*, **6:** 337.
23. Sultan, G. (1994) Buying an autoclave; *Practice Nursing*, 8–21 March: 21.
24. Department of the Environment (1991) *The Environment Protection Act 1990: Waste Management, the Duty of Care, a Code of Conduct.* DOE, London.
25. Health and Safety Executive prosecution (1988) Bradford Magistrates' Court.
26. *Journal of the Medical Defence Union* (1993) **9**(4): 79.

Further reading

British Medical Association (1990) *A Code of Practice for the Safe Disposal of Sharps*. BMA, London.

Useful addresses

FP Sales
28 Kelburne Road, Cowley, Oxford OX4 3SZ.
Telephone 0865-749333.

Williams Medical Supplies
Unit H6 Springhead Enterprise Park, Springhead,
Gravesend, Kent DA11 8DH.
Telephone 0474-535330. *Fax* 0474-335036
and
Unit 23 Heads of the Valley Industrial Estate
Rhymney, Gwent NP2 5RL.
Telephone 0685-844724. *Fax* 0685-844725.

Appendix 4.1
Examples of the clinical equipment needed in the nurses' rooms

Examination equipment

Examination couch, paper rolls, pillow, pillow covers, small blanket
Directable lamp
Accurate weighing scales, height measure, body mass index chart
Sphygmomanometer and stethoscope
Oral, rectal and low-reading thermometers
Auriscope with aural specula in all sizes
Pen-torch and tongue depressors
Spare batteries and bulbs
Eye chart
Tissues
Unsterile latex gloves
Examination jelly
Disposal bags and pedal bins

Clinical test equipment

Adult and low-reading peak flow meters and mouthpieces
Micro spirometer
Inhaler devices and medication for reversibility tests
Charts of normal values
Urinalysis test strips
Pregnancy tests
Sterile receptacles for collecting MSUs
Paediatric urine collecting bags
Blood glucose test strips, lancets and glucose meter
Injection trays, syringes, needles, vacuum system barrels, alcohol wipes, cotton wool balls, tourniquets, small adhesive plasters
Pathological specimen bottles, request forms, ESR stand
Sharps bins and yellow bags for clinical waste
Aylesbury spatulae, endocervical brushes, glass slides and fixative, carrying boxes
Sterile swabs and transport medium
Electrocardiogram machine
Screening audiometer
Doppler ultrasound
Smokelyser
Microscope (if needed)

Equipment for nursing procedures

Dressings

Sterile dressing packs, sterile and unsterile gauze squares
Normal saline solution, hydrogen peroxide solution
Non-adherent dressings
Hydrocolloid dressings – 10 × 10cm
Hydrogel sachets
Calcium alginate dressings – 5 × 5cm and 7.5 × 10cm
Semi-permeable film dressings
Skin closure strips (GP41)

Adhesive tapes

Hypoallergenic tape – 1.25mm and 2.5mm
Elastoplast tape – 2.5mm
Hypafix or *Mefix* paper backed tape – 2.5mm and 5mm

Bandages

Conforming bandages – 5cm, 7.5cm and 10cm
Cotton crepe bandages – 5cm, 7.5cm, 10cm and 15cm
Compression bandages – 10cm (if used)
Tubular bandages – e.g. *Tubegauz* sizes 01, 12 and 56
Triangular bandages

Miscellaneous

Range of plastic bowls for washing patients' legs, disinfecting nebuliser chambers, vomit bowl etc
Emollient creams e.g. *Diprobase, E45, Unguentum Merck*
Dressing scissors
Stitch cutters, staple and clip removers
Ring-cutter
Cold pack for soft-tissue injuries

Ear syringing

Auriscope and specula
Cape and towel
Jug for warm water
Noots tank or receiver
Pulsed water unit or ear syringe
Tissues

Minor surgery equipment

Autoclave, purified water, test strips
Disposable plastic aprons
Hibiscrub
Sterile surgeon's gloves
Xylocaine 1% – with, and without, Adrenaline
Ethyl chloride spray
Trolley
Sterile minor surgery packs or dressing packs
Gallipots
Povidone iodine or chlorhexidine skin cleanser
Scalpel handles and blades
Toothed and non-toothed dissecting forceps
Straight and curved artery forceps
Curette
Needle holders
Straight and curved scissors
Splinter forceps
Sinus forceps
Nail elevator
Specimen containers and formaldehyde solution
Cautery
Silver nitrate sticks
Sterile suture materials – catgut, nylon, silk – 3/0, 4/0, 5/0, 6/0 sizes
Liquid nitrogen, or aerosol freezer spray
Disposable plastic bags
Disposable plastic bags and bowl for soiled instruments, household gloves, washing up liquid
Lubricant for instruments
Household bleach/Presept granules (for blood spillage)

Injections

Stock injections as needed e.g. hydroxocobalamin, *Modecate, Depixol*, vaccines

Family planning and gynaecological equipment

Vaginal specula – virginal, small, medium, large and extra large Cusco's, and small Winterton's (with longer blades)
Sponge-holding forceps
Tissue forceps
Uterine sound
Long artery forceps
Long round-ended scissors
Emmett thread retriever

Range of sterile IUDs
Sanitary towels

Caps and diaphragms

Sizing rings
Range of practice caps and diaphragms
Diaphragm introducers
Spermicides for demonstration
Instruction leaflets

Injectables

Depo-Provera, Norethisterat

Demonstration samples for teaching

Contraceptive pills, condoms, IUDs and implants
Instruction leaflets

Appendix 4.2
Emergency equipment

Collapse

Injection tray, syringes, needles, swabs, and emergency drugs:

>   Adrenaline 1:1000 in 1ml for I/M use (see Fig. 7.4 for dosage)
>   Chlorpheniramine 10mg in 1ml for I/M or I/V use
>   Hydrocortisone sodium succinate 100mg for I/V or I/M use
>   Atropine sulphate 600mg in 1 ml for I/M or I/V use
>   Glucagon 1mg dose for I/M use
>   Dextrose 50% in 25ml for I/V use
>   Terbutyline (*Bricanyl*) 0.5mg in 1ml for I/M or slow I/V use
>   Prochlorperazine (*Stemetil*) 12.5mg in 1ml, and 25mg in 2ml for I/M use
>   Diazepam 10mg in 2ml for I/M or I/V use
>   Frusemide 400mg in 5ml for I/V use

Airways in range of sizes – infant to large adult
Adult and infant resuscitation masks and Ambu bag
Oxygen cylinder and giving set
Suction machine
Intravenous needles, giving set and normal saline infusion and/or plasma substitute
Defibrillator (not commonly kept in urban practices, but could be needed in remote districts)

Emergency asthma treatment

Nebuliser with adult and child's masks
Salbutamol 2.5 and 5mg nebules
Ipratropium bromide (*Atrovent*) nebules

Eye tray

Magnifying head lens (Loup)
Normal saline *Steripods*, for irrigation
Eye drops: Fluorescein 1%
            Amethocaine 1%
            Chloromycetin
            Tropicamide
            Mydrilate 0.5%
            Atropine sulphate 1%
Most of the eyedrops listed can be obtained in separate sterile *Minims*, which can be purchased from the local chemist or wholesaler.
Chloromycetin eye ointment

Non-filamented gauze swabs, and tissues
Eye bath
Sterile eye pads and microporous tape 1.25cm

Epistaxis tray

Nasal specula in a range of sizes
Nasal forceps
Scissors
Calcium alginate dressing (*Kaltostat*), ribbon gauze impregnated with bismuth and iodoform paraffin paste (BIPP), or *Sterispon* – a synthetic sponge which reabsorbs without having to be removed

Laryngeal tray

Xylocaine laryngeal spray
Head mirror and lamp
Methylated spirit lamp and matches
Tongue depressor
Laryngeal mirror
Nasal forceps
Throat forceps
Gauze swabs

Chapter 5
Nursing Procedures

Thoughtful preparation and skilled performance can minimise the discomfort caused by some nursing procedures. Even apparently routine tasks provide opportunities for health promotion and active listening to patients' concerns.

Injections

A variety of injections are given in general practice. (Specific injections are dealt with in the relevant chapters.) Nurses with district nursing and health visitor qualifications, who have had the additional training required, will soon be legally allowed to prescribe from the limited range of medicines and dressings in the Nurse Prescribers' Formulary[1]. However, injections must be prescribed by a doctor: either in the patient's records, on a separate authorisation form, or a prescription form (FP10). Routine immunisations may be given without a prescription, providing the arrangements and criteria for immunisation are covered by a protocol[2]. The standards of care should include the following points.

Organisation

The drugs and vaccines for injection must be stored as directed by the manufacturers.

Whenever possible, appointments should be available at suitable times. Patients who work will need flexible appointment times. Some immunisations may have to be given opportunistically in order to reach the specific targets. There should be an adequate supply of disposable syringes and needles, and sharps bins. Prefilled syringes are available for some vaccines and emergency drugs. Adrenaline should always be at hand in case of anaphylaxis.

Injection procedure

Any contraindications to an injection must be identified, and the patient referred to the doctor if necessary. If there is any doubt about the drug name, dosage, or route of administration the GP or a pharmacist should be consulted.

(Injection techniques are taught in pre-registration training and will not be described here.)

Patients should have all the information they require to give informed consent for the injection.

Nervous patients will be less likely to faint if they lie down to be injected. An intramuscular injection into the buttock can be given more safely when the patient is lying on a couch.

Young children may like a teddy bear to cuddle while being injected; as may a few adults! A badge or certificate of bravery, will console many children afterwards. Feeding seems to be the best pacifier for young infants, while a bright, musical toy will usually distract older babies. Anaesthetic cream (*Emla*) can be applied to the injection site half an hour before injection, for very nervous children, and those who require a large number of injections.

The injection should be prepared and administered according to the manufacturer's instructions. Advice may be needed on alternative routes of administration for patients with bleeding disorders, who should not be given intramuscular injections. The most appropriate needle should be selected for the injection method and size of the patient.

The needle must not be resheathed, as this is the most common cause of needle-stick injuries. The syringe and needle must be placed in a sharps bin immediately after use.

Records

A nurse could be legally responsible for any harm to a patient, if unable to prove the source of the product used[3]. Therefore records must be kept of the product name, dose, route of administration, manufacturer, batch number and expiry date. This applies to any medicine – not just injections. The site of injection should also be recorded, especially when more than one injection is given, in case of an adverse reaction to one of them.

The injection data may also be needed for immunisation targets or for a recall system for regular medication.

After injection

The nurse must observe the patient until satisfied that there are no immediate ill-effects from the injection. It is not possible to specify an exact time[4]. Some practice policies state a minimum time of 20 minutes. (See Chapter 7, *Emergency Situations.*)

Patients need information about possible side-effects and the action to take if they occur. The product data sheets list all the possible adverse reactions.

Patients receiving regular injections should know when to make the next appointment. A recall system may be needed for immunisations, or depot medication.

Wound care

Practice nurses are likely to encounter patients with a variety of wounds. The range of dressings can be bewildering and sales representatives produce convincing arguments for favouring their own products. A sound understanding of the principles of wound healing is necessary when selecting a dressing. A district wound care specialist will provide education and advice, and some health districts have product formularies, which can make the selection process easier.

Wound healing

There are three distinct phases of healing, although some overlap occurs between them:

- *Inflammation* – in response to the initial injury. A fibrin clot forms, to prevent further blood loss. Blood vessels in the vicinity of the wound become more permeable and leucocytes are attracted to the area to remove bacteria and debris by phagocytosis. (The normal inflammatory response, which causes slight redness around a wound, should not be mistaken for infection.)
- *Proliferation* – of cells and collagen. Fibroblasts produce collagen fibres, and buds of endothelial cells and capillaries grow into the wound space to form the delicate granulation tissue. Occasionally overgranulation can occur above the level of the surrounding skin.
- *Maturation* – as the wound heals. Epithelial cells migrate across the wound until it is covered. Collagen is broken down and remoulded over subsequent months to form a firmer scar. Keloid forms when there is an overproduction of collagen.

Wounds are often classified according to their appearance or stage of healing:

- *Necrotic wounds* – when devitalised tissue forms a dry, hard, black eschar, or a soft, grey slough. Surgical or chemical debridement is necessary.
- *Infected wounds* – when bacteria overcome the body's natural defences. There may be a purulent discharge and/or cellulitis present. Systemic antibiotics may be needed if infection is confirmed by microbiological swab results. All wounds become colonised by bacteria, but are not necessarily 'infected'.
- *Clean wounds* – are those without slough or infection. They may be superficial or deep. The skin margins of incisions may be drawn together to reduce the gap to be bridged. Wider wounds heal by granulation.

Necrotic or infected tissue delays healing and must be treated. Wounds usually heal more quickly in the warm, moist environment created by an occlusive dressing because the epithelial cells can migrate across the wound rather than growing downwards under a scab[5].

Dressings

Unfortunately there are many products available in hospitals which are denied to staff working in the community. Where a good case can be made for including such items on the *Drug Tariff* nurses should lobby the Department of Health to get the items included.

The dressing range available on prescription includes:

Sterile dressing packs which open to provide a sterile field and contain a hand-towel/paper drape, four cotton wool balls, four gauze swabs and a dressing pad. The packs are expensive and may not be needed for minor dressings. Packs of five sterile gauze swabs, or 100 unsterile swabs are available.

Normal saline (*Normasol, Steripods*) as single-use 25ml units for cleansing wounds. Antiseptics can damage fragile granulation tissue and are generally contraindicated[6].

Enzyme preparations (*Varidase*) can be used to debride necrotic tissue. The preparation is expensive, but it can last a little longer mixed with *KY jelly* and stored in the refrigerator.

Hydrocolloid dressings (*Comfeel, Granuflex, Tegasorb*) are waterproof adhesive wafers which combine with exudate from a wound to form a gel; useful for desloughing wounds and promoting granulation. Hydrocolloid paste can be used in deep wounds and sinuses.

They can sometimes cause overgranulation if used too long. The liquid which forms under the wafer can be mistaken for pus. The offensive odour of the liquid, and leakage can distress patients. Skin maceration can occur if there is excessive exudate.

Hydrogels (*Intrasite gel*) a soft gel packaged in sachets, which can be applied directly to a wound and covered with an occlusive film or secondary dressing. The gel helps to rehydrate wounds and create the optimum conditions for healing. It has a range of uses similar to hydrocolloids.

Calcium alginate dressings (*Kaltostat, Sorbsan*) are made of an extract of seaweed spun and woven into soft mats. Useful as a haemostatic and for absorbing exudate. Can be moistened with saline and used under occlusive films or other secondary dressings. They can be removed from wounds by saline irrigation. The dressings sometimes stick fast, but soaking with saline will work, with patience.

Cavity packing material is also produced, but is not available on prescription.

Polyurethane foam (*Lyofoam*) absorbs exudate through the non-adherent contact layer into the foam backing; has many uses as a primary dressing. Can be used under compression bandages, and as a light, comfortable dressing for arterial ulcers. The foam can be cut easily and makes a good dressing after toe-nail surgery. It is useful for controlling overgranulation.

Semi-permeable film dressings (*Bioclusive, Opsite, Tegaderm*) can be used to secure a dressing or to provide a warm, moist environment for clean, superficial wounds. Also useful for keeping enzymatic preparations moist.

Some patients are allergic to the adhesive. Skin can be damaged if the film is pulled away. It should be lifted and stretched off the skin.

Non-adherent dressings (*N-A Dressing, Tricotex*) are thin wound contact dressings designed to be non-adherent, but are often difficult to remove. Can be used for venous ulcers under compression bandages. Also useful for minor burns, used with silver sulphadiazine cream (*Flamazine*). Secondary dressings are needed.

Impregnated gauze (*Paratulle, Bactigras*) have limited uses. Paraffin gauze might be used occasionally on skin graft sites or as a carrier for *Flamazine* cream for burns. Allergic reactions can occur.

Strapping and bandages may be applied to secure a dressing, to give support or provide compression to an underlying structure.

Adhesive tape can be used to secure dressings, or for neighbour-strapping injured fingers and toes. Many people are allergic to zinc oxide adhesive and it can be difficult to remove.

Microporous tape (*Micropore*) is light, hypoallergenic and easy to remove. Some patients can be allergic to the adhesive. The tape is used to secure dressings, but it does not stretch as the body moves. Strips of sterile microporous tape (*Steri-strips*) can be used to close minor incisions.

Paper-backed tape (*Hypafix*, *Mefix*) is not available on prescription, but is a light, stretchable fixative, which if used sparingly, is not too expensive to buy.

Conforming bandages (*Kling*, *Slinky*) are light, loosely woven bandages for securing dressings. The edges of Kling can cut into oedematous tissue if applied too tightly, and Slinky has elastic fibres which if overextended can cause oedema above and below the bandage.

Tubular bandages (*Tubefast*, *Tubegauz*,) come in a range of sizes, and can hold dressings in place, or be used under bandages to protect sensitive skin. The small sizes are useful for dressing fingers and toes. *Tubegauz* applicators are available.

Tubigrip in sizes B to G provides support for soft tissue injuries. It is meant to be used double, but single layers are useful for keeping dressings and bandages in place. Special measuring tapes can be obtained from the manufacturers for assessing the size needed. Shaped Tubigrip gives firmer support, but is not available on prescription.

Crepe bandages can be used to secure dressings or to provide support for soft tissue injuries.

Paste bandages (*PB7*, *Icthapaste*, *Quinoband*) can be used in conjunction with compression bandages to treat venous ulcers. Severe allergies can develop to some of the constituents. A skin test is recommended before applying a paste bandage.

Elastic crepe bandages (*Elastocrepe*) provide support, but give insufficient compression and quickly lose their elasticity. Tuition and practice is needed to get the correct amount of extension when applying them.

Compression bandages (*Setopress*, *Tensopress*) give a much greater level of compression and can be washed several times and reused. Markings on the bandages indicate how far to stretch them. Severe ischaemic damage can be caused by inappropriate use. Doppler ultrasound or arterial assessment is needed first.

Compression hosiery can be prescribed for individual patients: men and women. There are three classes of compression:

- Class I gives the least compression.
- Class II gives the moderate compression needed for most patients in general practice.
- Class III is for very firm compression.

The stockings can have closed or open toes and be knee or thigh length. Black support hose are available for men, and made to measure hose can be prescribed for patients with unusual measurements. Stocking aids can be obtained via the occupational therapist for patients who have difficulty putting on support hose.

General assessment of the patient

Wound care entails much more than applying dressings. A full assessment is needed. The factors to consider include:

Age

Elderly patients have slower rates of growth and repair, less collagen and elasticity in the skin, and may have impaired circulation. The immune system can also be less effective. Care is needed to avoid damaging fragile skin with adhesives or tight bandages.

Mobility

Patients who are not very mobile are more likely to develop oedema, or to fall. Referrals for physiotherapy or occupational therapy may be needed to help to improve mobility. Housebound patients may need to be referred to the district nurse for treatment.

Nutritional state

Obesity can contribute to reduced mobility and make bandaging difficult. Malnourished or cachexic patients can lack the vitamins and minerals needed for wound healing. Patients may need information about healthy eating. Those who are unable to eat a healthy diet may require food supplements or to see to a dietician. Protein intake can be checked by liver function tests (albumin levels).

Medical condition

The general medical condition can influence the progress of any wound. Anaemia, diabetes, rheumatoid arthritis, immunosuppression, and cardio-pulmonary disease can all contribute to the development or continuation of tissue damage. A doctor should be consulted when necessary.

The advocates of holistic care maintain that the immune system can be boosted by a positive attitude to any disease process. Alternative therapies reduce stress and induce well-being, and so may assist wound healing[7].

Psychological state

The patient's motivation should be assessed. Patients may lack the energy or inclination to care for themselves properly, or they may have self-inflicted injuries. Counselling and/or antidepressant therapy may be needed.

Social situation

Lonely patients have been suspected sometimes of exacerbating their wounds to maintain contact with the nurse[8]. Referrals may be made to social services or voluntary agencies to arrange other contacts.

Smoking

Smoking reduces the amount of oxygen available to the tissues, and increases the damage to small blood vessels[9].

Alcohol intake

A high alcohol intake can adversely affect the nutritional state and cause damage to the liver and kidneys.

Pain

Pain may limit mobility or affect sleep. Analgesics might be needed, and the choice of dressing can be influenced if the wound is very painful.

The assessment and treatment of the wound

The wound assessment should include: the type, size, stage of healing, amount of exudate, and any complicating factors.

Measurements of the wound will provide an objective scale against which to judge progress. Tracing over a double plastic film is a quick, easy method which allows the top layer to be kept free from contamination by the wound. Photographs also provide a good reference. A ruler should be included in the picture to show the scale.

Choosing a dressing

See Fig. 5.1. Things to consider:

● *practical issues* – getting shoes on, bathing, frequency of dressing changes, patient compliance,

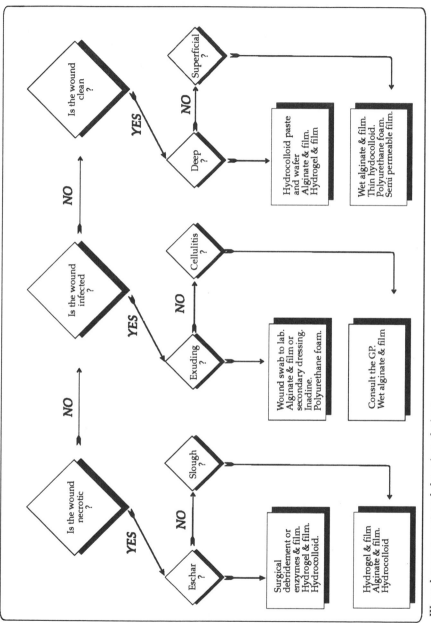

Fig. 5.1 Wound assessment and dressing choices.

- *aesthetic factors* – how the dressings looks, feels, smells,
- *cost* – can be important, but should not deter the use of the most suitable product.

Wound care is most effective if the patient is involved in planning the treatment and lifestyle changes necessary to promote healing. Advice may be sought from a wound care adviser if a wound poses particular difficulties. The possibility of malignancy should always be considered if a wound fails to heal or is recurrent.

Leg ulcers

Leg ulcers, often painful and debilitating to patients, use vast resources in manpower and dressings annually. The correct diagnosis of the ulcer type is essential before treatment is started.

Arterial ulcers

These result from ischaemia due to arterial occlusion; often caused by arterioslerosis. Minor trauma may cause an ulcer to develop, and the tissue breaks down as a result of impaired supply of oxygen and nutrients. Smoking exacerbates the problem.

Recognition

- *position of the ulcer* – often below the ankle,
- *appearance* – often well-demarcated, deep, with a pale base, necrosis and absence of healthy granulation tissue. The skin around the ulcer may be shiny and dry, and the toe-nails thickened,
- *pain* – particularly at night, often severe,
- *foot pulses* – may be absent or diminished. (Experience is needed to locate foot pulses. NOT AN ACCURATE INDICATOR).

Assessment of arterial blood-flow by Doppler ultrasound is more objective, and early referral for arteriography, if appropriate.

Aims of treatment

- to reduce pain
- to assist healing
- to prevent further tissue damage.

Treatment	Rationale
Ensure the patient has adequate analgesia and knows when to take it.	Ischaemic ulcers can be very painful.
Identify any contributing medical conditions.	Diabetes, rheumatoid arthritis, anaemia and malignancy may contribute to ischaemic ulcers.
Refer for systemic antibiotics.	If the wound is infected.
Dressings, e.g. *Lyofoam*, *Intrasite gel*.	For lightness and comfort and ease of removal, and to encourage healing.
Encourage cessation of smoking.	To prevent further vascular damage and improve O_2 supply to the tissues.
Avoid compression.	To avoid compromising the circulation further.

Surgery may be indicated to try and improve the blood-flow for patients with ischaemia. In extreme cases amputation can become necessary.

Venous ulcers

These result from inadequacy of the venous drainage of the legs. Incompetent valves in the perforator veins allow a back-flow and increased venous pressure in the superficial veins.

Recognition

- *skin condition* -- varicose eczema, brown discolouration caused by the breakdown of red blood cells in the tissues,
- *ulcer position* – commonest in the gaiter area, the pre-tibial and anteromedial supramalleolar areas,
- *appearance* – superficial with uneven edges and some granulation tissue,
- *oedema* – due to venous insuffiency; often exacerbated by reduced mobility,
- *pain* – infected ulcers may be painful, but often patients are pain-free.

Aims of treatment

- To improve the venous return and reduce stagnation in the tissues of the affected leg.
- To provide clear information and encouragement to enable the

patient to participate in the treatment and to maintain his/her legs in their optimum condition after healing has occurred.

Treatment	Rationale
Wash the leg ulcer with warm water.	To remove debris without damaging the wound surface or cooling the wound.
Apply a flat, non-irritant, non-adherent dressing or a hydrocolloid wafer.	To prevent indentation of surrounding skin and allow removal of the dressing without damage to healing tissues.
Pad smoothly with gauze or other absorbent material.	To absorb exudate and protect bony prominences.
Apply graduated compression by bandaging or compression hosiery. (Needs to be sustained at approximately 40 mmHg at the ankle[10].	To reverse venous hypertension without compromising the arterial circulation.
Advise elevation of the foot above the level of the hip when resting.	To reduce oedema by using gravity.
Teach suitable ankle exercises. (Dorsi- and plantar flexing feet, circular movements of the ankles.)	To aid the venous return by action of the calf-muscle pump.
Prevent a recurrence by good skin-care, compression hosiery and early treatment of injury.	Patients who understand their condition can take responsibility for their legs and seek help early.

Compression bandaging cannot be learned from a book. Expert tuition and practice are needed.

Mixed ulcers

Some patients have mixed ulcers caused by both arterial and venous insufficiency. Compression must be avoided where there is any risk to the arterial blood flow.

Ear syringing

This procedure is usually carried out by practice nurses for the removal of excessive ear-wax. Warm olive oil, sodium bicarbonate or proprietary softening drops should be recommended for use three days before syringing.

Occasionally patients may require ear syringing to remove a foreign body or debris. The protocol should specify the circumstances under which patients may self-refer for treatment, and the contraindications to syringing. A patient with a history of earache, discharge or perforation should not have his/her ears syringed without an initial assessment by the doctor.

Equipment needed

Lamp
Auriscope and range of specula
Ear syringe or electric pulsed water unit (the syringe should be lubricated just enough to move freely with pressure)
Noots tank or receiver
Plastic cape and towel
Jug of warm water
Tissues

Action	Rationale
Arrange the patient's chair and position the lamp.	So the nurse can move freely and have a clear view of the patient's ears.
Examine the ears with the auriscope.	To assess the suitability for syringing.
Explain the procedure to the patient. Use diagrams and demonstrate the equipment.	To ensure co-operation while syringing is being performed. Patients can be nervous – especially if they have not had their ears syringed before.
Explain that it should not cause pain, and to report any discomfort so the procedure can be stopped at once.	Some people might not want to make a fuss, so could experience pain but not mention it and suffer trauma to the ear.
Use water at body temperature.	Extremes of temperature cause dizziness.
Protect the patient's clothes with the cape and towel, and the nurse's with a disposable apron.	Water will run out, and can splash back while the ear is being syringed.
Ask the patient to hold the Noots tank or receiver slightly below the ear.	To catch the water as it runs out without pressing below the auditory canal.
Draw up water into the ear syringe and holding with the nozzle upwards, expel any air. Or run the water through the tubing of the pulsed water unit.	To ensure an even flow of water without air bubbles. To expel any cold water remaining in the tubing.

Make sure the nozzle is well-secured (especially with a pulsed water unit).	It can damage the auditory canal or even perforate the drum if it flies off under the pressure of the water.
Hold the pinna with the non-dominant hand and gently pull the pinna backwards and upwards (downwards if a child).	To help to straighten the auditory canal without pinching and to ensure that the ear is held steady so no injury will occur.
Allow the patient to feel the water temperature on the ear.	To make sure there is no sudden movement if the patient is surprised.
Direct the water to the top and back of the auditory meatus using a controlled pressure. (Fig. 5.2).	To avoid direct pressure on the eardrum. The water should run behind the wax or foreign body and lift it out. Excess pressure can perforate the drum.
Do not jam the nozzle tightly into the meatus.	It might cause trauma to the ear.
Inspect the ears frequently with the auriscope during the procedure and afterwards.	To check progress and ensure that no trauma is being caused. To ensure that the ear looks normal.
Offer the patient a tissue.	To dry around the ear.
Refer a patient with any abnormality of the ear to the GP.	Medical treatment may be necessary.
Ensure that the patient understands how to care for his/her ears and how to avoid trauma.	Many people think they should clean their ears with cotton buds. This can cause impaction of the wax and damage the lining of the auditory canal.

Patients with impacted wax may need to use softening drops for a longer period, or be referred back to the GP. Very gentle water pressure should be used to remove debris after treatment for an ear infection.

Eye treatments

(See Chapter 7, *Foreign bodies* and Chapter 8, *Eye conditions.*)

Patients may ask to see the practice nurse with conditions they think too trivial to bother the doctor. Nurses are advised to err on the side of caution and refer to the GP, when in any doubt about dealing with eye conditions.

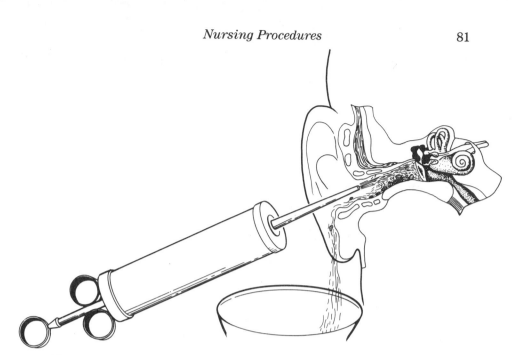

Fig. 5.2 Ear syringing.

The principles of eye care are:

Action	Rationale
Avoid using antiseptic spray on the hands.	Can cause irritation to the patient's eyes.
Ensure there is a good light source.	To be able to assess the eye properly and avoid injury during any eye treatment.
Avoid shining the light directly into the eye.	The patient might have photophobia.
Tell the patient what is being done.	To avoid sudden movements which could injury the eye.
Inspect the eye for signs of infection, allergy or injury.	To detect any problem and to ensure the correct treatment is given.
Enquire about the patient's vision.	In case of any abnormality which needs investigation.
Clean the lids thoroughly with normal saline or cooled, boiled water. Use each swab once only and discard it.	If necessary – to remove any discharge. To avoid spreading infection to the other eye.

Hold the dropper, or nozzle of the ointment tube about 1cm away from the eye. (Fig. 5.3).

To avoid damage to the cornea and to prevent contaminating the tube or dropper.
Drops from too great a height can be painful.

Instil drops into the outer corner of the lower lid.

Drops into the punctal end will drain straight into the nose.

Make sure that patients understand how to continue their treatment at home, and under which circumstances to seek medical help. Stress the importance of hand hygiene and of keeping separate face towels – especially when a patient has conjunctivitis.

Assisting with minor surgery

The advantages to patients of the growth of minor surgery in general practice include reduced waiting times for treatment and a more personal service in a familiar environment. Many doctors and nurses enjoy the chance to extend their professional skills.

The standards of care required for performing minor surgery in general practice must include: the control of infection, the comfort and safety of the patient and the ability to deal with emergency situations.

The practice nurse's role

Preparation of the environment

The practice nurse has a responsibility for ensuring the high standard of cleanliness in the room used for minor surgery. The couch and lamp should be positioned to allow free access to the operation site. A comfortable room temperature is needed. Curtains or blinds should be adjusted to give privacy to patients.

Preparation of the equipment

Trolleys should be cleaned with soap and water and dried with paper towels[11]. If CSSD packs are not available the instruments have to be sterilised and laid between sterile paper sheets, but trolleys must not be laid up more than three hours in advance because of the risk of contamination with micro-organisms[12].

Preparation of the patient

Most people will experience some apprehension. Practice nurses can

---

READ THIS NOTE BEFORE USING YOUR MEDICINE

NAME OF PREPARATION, DOSAGE INSTRUCTIONS   PATIENTS NAME

PRESCRIBING DOCTOR   DATE

THE USE OF EYE OINTMENT

1. Wash hands before use.
2. When using a new tube for the first time,
   squeeze out a 1/2" (about 1 cm) strip and throw it away
3. To use:
   (a) Tilt the head back slightly
   (b) With the lower lid turned down, gently apply a strip of ointment
       about 1/2" (or 1 cm) long to the inner surface of the lid.
   (c) Close the eye, and gently massage the lids for a few seconds.
   (d) Remove any surplus ointment with a clean tissue
   (e) Vision may be blurred after applying the medication.
       Do not drive or operate machinery until vision is clear.

   if you find this difficult, it may be easier for someone else to do this for you.

4. Always replace the cap, and keep the tube in a cool place.
5. Avoid letting the nozzle of the tube touch the surface of the eye,
   or the lashes or table tops etc.
6. NEVER share your eye ointment with other people.
7. Discard any remainder when the treatment is finished, or after four weeks.

Further advice may be obtained from your pharmacist or doctor

Pharmacist's Name: Telephone Number

Address:

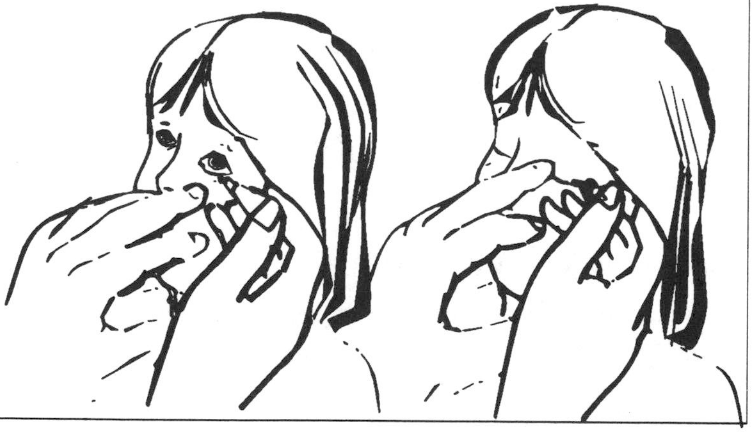

Fig. 5.3 Instructions for the use of eye ointment. (Reproduced with the permission of Barrie and Jenkins *The Action and Uses of Ophthalmic drugs.*)

help by ensuring patients receive a clear explanation of what to expect, and by encouraging the use of simple relaxation techniques. Patients commonly request to have moles and other skin lesions removed but are then surprised to learn that they will have a scar. Even if the doctor has obtained written consent, the nurse can reinforce the information given.

Each patient should be asked to remove clothing as necessary to make sure the operation site is accessible. Clothing not removed should be protected from any possible blood trickles. Even small lesions can be surprisingly vascular. If the operation site is on the scalp some hair may need to be trimmed, or it may be possible just to tape hair out of the way.

During the operation

The main responsibilities of the nurse are to comfort and observe the patient during the minor operation, and to assist the doctor as needed. For example, by checking the local anaesthetic, opening sterile packs, receiving specimens for histology, and possibly assisting with suturing. The nurse will usually dress the wound and select the appropriate fixative.

After the operation

The patient may need time to recover before leaving the surgery. The nurse should ensure that the patient is able to get home safely and understands how to care for the wound and when to return. Written advice sheets can be useful because verbal instructions are easily forgotten. The stress experienced by patients undergoing what can seem to be trivial procedures, should never be underestimated.

Clearing up often falls to the nurse. Although the safe disposal of sharps is the responsibility of the person who used them, extreme caution is needed in case any have been overlooked. Items left on the bottom of trolleys can be hazardous to children, so trolleys must be cleared completely.

Basic minor operation trolley

Each doctor may have favourite instruments but a basic set usually comprises:

- scalpel handle
- toothed dissecting forceps
- plain dissecting forceps
- curette

- artery forceps
- needle holder
- scissors

Plus a sterile gallipot.
  Also needed are:

- disposable apron
- *Hibiscrub*
- sterile surgeon's gloves
- local anaesthetic
- syringes and needles
- chlorhexidine and alcohol skin prep
- scalpel blade
- specimen container and formaldehyde solution
- suture materials
- dressings and fixative.

A silver nitrate stick or cautery may also be required.

The doctors' preferences will determine the equipment for specific procedures but some of the extra instruments and equipment include the following.

Removal of sebacious cysts

Instruments: Curved scissors and mosquito forceps to dissect out a cyst and keep the capsule intact.

Incision of abscesses

Equipment: Ethylchloride spray (local anaesthetic). A wound swab and transport medium for microbiology.

Instruments: Sinus forceps or a probe.

Dressing: Alginate strip for light packing.

Note: Although it is good practice to ensure all patients undergoing minor surgery have had a routine urinalysis, boils, abscesses or carbuncles should raise particular suspicions about diabetes mellitus.

Ingrowing toe-nails

Removal of an ingrowing toe-nail may be necessary if conservative treatment or wedge resection is unsuccessful. Advice and information on footcare may help to prevent a recurrence.

Equipment: *Plain lignocaine* 1% as local anaesthetic for a ring-block because the vasoconstriction caused by adrenaline can cause gangrene of a digit.

Instruments: a nail elevator and sturdy, pointed scissors.

Dressings: need to be easily removed without causing pain e.g. polyurethane foam, calcium alginate, or hydrocolloid.

Skin tags

Small skin tags can be tied tightly with suture silk, which causes them to drop off after a few days.

Note: as this method creates a small area of necrosis, check anti-tetanus cover and offer injection if necessary.

Warts and verrucae

If proprietary treatments, (*Cuplex, Salatac*), are unsuccessful, cryotherapy using liquid nitrogen or aerosol freezing solution (*Histofreezer*) may work. Practice nurses can develop expertise in this field, but must be taught to perform the treatments safely. Some warts require surgical excision.

Insertion of inter-uterine device (IUD)

See Chapter 12 for further details. The following equipment is required.

Sterile equipment

- Cusco speculum
- long artery forceps
- sponge-holding forceps
- volsellum forceps
- uterine sound
- long round-ended scissors
- gallipot.

Plus: sterile gloves, cleansing solution, thread retriever, selection of IUDs, KY jelly, sanitary towel, emergency tray.

Unsterile demonstration IUDs are useful for teaching patients about the devices. A practice nurse needs to understand the insertion procedure in order to explain it to patients, and assist the doctor when necessary.

Procedure

- The patient should have an empty bladder, and remove tights and pants. Then be made comfortable on the couch and covered with a small blanket.
- The doctor performs a bimanual examination, to identify any pelvic abnormalities.
- A vaginal speculun is inserted to visualise the cervix. The nurse may need to adjust the light.
- The cervix is cleansed with a swab moistened with a cleansing solution held in the sponge-holding forceps.
- If the patient has an IUD in situ, it is removed with the long forceps, and thread retriever if needed.
- The tissue forceps may be attached, to hold the cervix steady.
- The uterine sound is inserted through the cervix to assess the length and position of the uterine cavity.
- The nurse opens the outer pack of the IUD selected and drops the contents onto the sterile field.
- The doctor prepares the device and introducer and inserts it through the cervix into the uterine cavity.
- The introducer is withdrawn, leaving the IUD in situ.
- The threads are cut with the long scissors.
- The speculum is removed.

On rare occasions, a patient may suffer cervical shock, so the emergency tray is needed. A patient with epilepsy could have a seizure precipitated by the insertion of an IUD[13]. The nursing care of a patient having an IUD inserted is covered in Chapter 12 (*Sexual Health*).

Suggestions for evaluation and research

- Devise a study to compare two dressing products for comfort, healing times and cost.
- Audit the patients having ear syringing:
    - (a) how effectively have softening drops been used?

    (b)   How many times have drops been used?

    (c)   What seems to be the optimum time for using them?

● Audit any healing problems or infected wounds following minor surgery. Consider if/how they might have been prevented.

References

1.   Great Britain, Parliament (1992) *Medicinal Products: Prescription by Nurses etc Act 1992.* HMSO, London.

2.   United Kingdom Central Council for Nurses, Midwives and Health Visitors (1992) *Standards for the Administration of Medicines.* UKCC, London.

3.   Department of Trade and Industry (1987) *Guide to the Consumer Protection Act 1987: Product Liability and Safety Provisions.* DTI, London.

4.   DOH, Welsh Office, Scottish Office Home and Health Department, DHSS (Northern Ireland) (1992) *Immunisation against Infectious Disease:* 4.8.1. HMSO, London.

5.   Winter, G. (1971) Healing of skin wounds and the influence of dressings on the repair process, in Harkin, K. (Ed) *Surgical Dressings and Wound Healing.* Proceedings of a symposium in July 1970, Crosby and Lockwood.

6.   Leaper, D., Cameron, S. and Lancaster, J. (1987) Antiseptic solutions; *Community Outlook,* April: 30–32.

7.   Richardson, J. (1992) The holistic model; *Journal of District Nursing,* **10**(8): 22, 24.

8.   Wise, G. (1986) The social ulcer; *Nursing Times,* **82**(21): 47–49.

9.   Siana, J. (1992) The effect of smoking on tissue function; *Journal of Wound Care,* **1**(1): 37–39.

10. Moffat, C. (1992) Compression bandaging – the state of the art; *Journal of Wound Care,* **1**(1): 45–50.

11. Thomson, G. and Bullock, D. (1992) To clean, or not to clean; *Nursing Times,* **88**, 19 August: 66–68.

12. British Medical Association (1989) *A Code of Practice for Sterilisation of Instuments and Control of Cross-Infection.* BMA, London.

13. Royal College of Nursing (1991) *Family Planning Manual for Nurses.* RCN, London.

Further reading

David, J. (1986) *Wound Management – a Comprehensive Guide to Dressings and Healing.* Dunitz, London.

Morison, M. (1992) *A Colour Guide to the Nursing Management of Wounds.* Wolfe, London.

Morison, M. *A Colour Guide to the Assessment and Management of Leg Ulcers.* Wolfe, London.

Centre for Medical Education (1992) *The Wound Programme.* Centre for Medical Education, Dundee.
Stilwell, B. (1992) *Skills Update.* Macmillan Magazines, London.

Useful addresses

The Wound Care Society
PO Box 263, Northampton NN3 4UJ.
Telephone 0604-784696.

Tissue Viability Society
Odstock Hospital, Salisbury SP2 8OJ.
Telephone 0722-336262 Ex 4057.

Chapter 6
Diagnostic and Screening Tests

A practice nurse may undertake a range of investigative and screening procedures, either at the request of a GP, or directly initiated by the nurse. The standards of care for individual procedures should cover the following areas:.

Nurse education

Some skills can be learned within the practice, but when necessary, many departments of district general hospitals will provide specialist training. Phlebotomy, electrocardiography, and screening audiometry can be learned this way.

Expert tuition and practice under supervision are needed for cervical screening. In-house training is not always adequate[1]. Education in cervical screening is provided through family planning and Marie Curie courses, and there may also be local arrangements for ensuring the quality of cervical smears.

Protocols

Many practice nurses have the authority to test for rubella antibodies, serum lipids, glucose etc. There is a cost implication with most investigations; therefore decisions need to be made about who should be offered particular tests, and when the doctor should be consulted. Some programmes for cervical cytology are run almost entirely by practice nurses. There should be clear guidelines on when to refer patients to the GP.

Informed consent

Investigations must not be carried out without the patient's consent. Many tests can only be performed correctly if the patient knows what to expect and can co-operate. Tests for HIV antibodies must not be performed until the patient has been counselled fully and has decided to have the test[2].

Health education

Patients undergoing any sort of test are likely to be concerned about some aspect of their health. Most situations present a chance for health promotion, if sensitively handled. For example – patients frequently express half-joking hopes that 'clean' equipment is being used. Such expressions of concern offer a way of discussing worries about HIV infection openly.

The prevention of death from coronary heart disease is part of the nurse's health promotion role. A patient attending for an ECG, even if only for medical insurance purposes, is likely to be interested in his/her heart; so a discussion of the lifestyle factors likely to affect the heart can be initiated, if it seems appropriate.

Emergency procedures

Familiarity is needed with the procedures for dealing with needle-stick injuries and blood spillage and for coping with a patient who collapses for any reason.

Records and management of specimens

Pathology forms must be completed accurately and the specimen containers labelled with the patient's identification details. The practice requires a foolproof system for recording specimens sent for testing and results received. Samples should be placed in specimen bags before despatch to the laboratory. The Post Office has regulations requiring the secure packaging of any specimens sent by post[3]. Biohazard stickers may still be requested by laboratory staff on specimen bottles and forms of patients known to be at high risk of infectious diseases such as hepatitis B; although all specimens should be considered as potentially hazardous.

The laboratory should be consulted if there is doubt about a specimen which cannot be despatched the same day. Some tests give false results if delayed. Urine can be kept in a refrigerator at 4°C overnight. This delay should be noted on the form. Swabs in transport medium can be kept in a cool place, but should not be put in the fridge.

All tests and their results must be entered in the patient's records. The patient must know how he/she will be notified of the result(s). Some investigations take longer than others; so a patient required to telephone for results needs to know how many tests were performed.

Laboratory tests

A good relationship with the local laboratory staff is worth cultivating. Most pathology departments will supply a list of tests, giving the amounts of sample material needed, the type of specimen bottle and any special requirements like timing, or diet.

Blood tests

Requirements

Syringes and needles or vacuum system needles and holders
Sample tubes and pathology forms
Arm cushion with protective cover
Tourniquet and/or sphygmomanometer and cuff
Unsterile latex gloves
Alcohol wipes and cotton wool balls
Small adhesive plasters/ hypoallergenic tape

Action	Rationale
(The variations in technique are marked S for syringe and V for vacuum system.)	
Give an anxious patient the opportunity to lie down.	Recumbent patients will be less likely to faint.
Or: seat the patient where the arm can be supported. Use a small arm pillow if necessary.	To make sure the vein can be accessed easily.
S Select a large enough syringe.	For all the tests wanted.
V Attach the double-ended needle to the holder.	Vacuum tubes can be attached once the needle is in the vein.
If the rolled up sleeve is tight ask the patient to remove the garment.	Tight clothing above the elbow will contribute to haematoma formation after the needle is withdrawn.
Remember – most patients have TWO arms. Make sure the best site is chosen.	There can be marked differences in the accessibility of veins.

Apply the tourniquet above the elbow. If a suitable vein is still not visible or palpable, a sphygmomanometer and cuff inflated to approximately 80mm Hg can be more effective.

To distend the vein in the antecubital fossa without affecting the arterial blood flow.

Put on the latex gloves.

For protection against blood-borne infections.

Cleanse the skin and allow the alcohol to dry.

To destroy bacteria and avoid stinging at the puncture site.

Insert the needle at an appropriate angle and keep it still once in situ. (Fig. 6.1).

Depending on the depth of the vein. Too steep an angle might cause the needle tip to pass right through the vein.

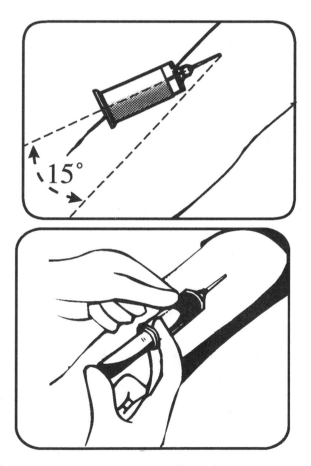

Fig. 6.1 Venepuncture using a vacutainer. (Reproduced with the permission of Becton Dickinson UK Ltd.)

S Withdraw the blood steadily, using gentle traction on the syringe piston*.	Too fast an action can haemolyse cells, too slow collection may allow the blood to coagulate.
V Attach each vacuum tube in turn keeping the needle steady. Use in order: (1) plain tubes (2) coagulation tube (3) other tubes with addititives.	Depending on the type of samples needed. To reduce the risk of contamination with anti-coagulants when clotted samples are needed.
Release the tourniquet.	Once blood flows into the first tube.
Gently mix the contents as each tube is removed.	If unclotted samples are needed.
Remove the last tube from the needle.	To avoid trauma to the vein.
S Release the tourniquet.	To relieve the pressure on the vein.
Place a cotton wool ball over the puncture site and withdraw the needle. Ask the patient to maintain firm pressure for 1–2 minutes, with the arm flat, not bent.	Extravasion of blood from the puncture site can cause bruising.
Do not resheath the needle.	This is the most common cause of needle-stick injuries.
S Remove the needle very carefully before filling the sample bottles.	Squirting blood through the needle will damage blood cells and affect test results.
S Fill the bottles to the required level.	Precise quantities of blood may be needed.
Dispose of needles, holders, and syringes into a sharps bin immediately after use.	To prevent infection and needle-stick injury.
S If other than a clotted sample required, gently mix the contents without shaking.	Anti-coagulant substances in the bottles need to be well mixed, without damaging the blood cells.
Cover the puncture site with a small adhesive plaster or use hypo-allergenic tape.	To prevent infection and any blood leaking onto the patient's sleeve.
Make sure the patient knows when and how to get the result of tests.	To ensure an abnormal result is not overlooked.
Complete the pathology forms and recheck the specimen labels.	Unlabelled specimens will not be processed.

* Note – the tourniquet should be released before collecting a blood sample for calcium levels[4].

Urine tests

Urine for microbiology

Midstream specimen of urine (MSU)

This test is meant to identify any organisms causing infection inside the urinary tract. Hence the need to collect specimens which are uncontaminated by skin and perineal flora. The perineal area should be washed and a specimen obtained after the urine flow has started. A sterile jug can be used if the patient cannot pass the specimen directly in the sample container.

Discussing the collection of an MSU also provides an opportunity to educate the patient about urinary infection and ways of preventing re-infection.

Clean catch specimen of urine

When a midstream urine specimen cannot be obtained, or is not necessary, the urine can be voided into a clean container. Special collection bags with an adhesive flange can be attached to the genital area of infants. The bags are expensive, but small quantities can be purchased from mail-order firms such as FP Sales.

Urine for cytology

Malignant cells in the urinary tract can be detected in urine samples. The patient should be instructed to void most of the urine and collect the sample (10–20ml) towards the end of the stream.

First-catch urine for chlamydia (Male patients only)

This method is more acceptable and can provide more reliable results than urethral swabs for chlamydia. The man should be asked not to empty his bladder for at least two hours. Then the first 20ml of urine should be collected in a sterile container.

24 hour urine collections

Large plastic containers and instruction sheets for collecting 24 hour specimens can be obtained from the laboratory. The containers for VMA analysis contain acid as a preservative and need safe storage.

Cervical smears (See Chapter 13, *Women's Health*)

The success of cervical screening depends on two factors:

(1)   ensuring that women attend,
(2)   obtaining adequate smears.

Practice nurses can help on both counts; by educating women about the need for screening and by learning to take good smears gently and sympathetically. *Warning:* this procedure cannot be learned from a book; the following is only intended as a reminder.

Requirements

Couch and adjustable light
Unsterile latex gloves
Glass microscope slide and pencil
Vaginal specula in range of sizes
Water-soluble lubricant (KY jelly)
Aylesbury spatula, and cervical brush (if in protocol)
Carbowax fixative
Tissues
Slide carrier
Cytology request form

Action	Rationale
Explain the procedure and answer any questions.	To make sure the patient knows what to expect.
Check the details with the patient and complete the cytology form.	To aid the cytologist's interpretation and ensure the patient is notified of the result.
Enquire about the patient's menstrual cycle and any abnormal symptoms.	Smears should be taken mid-cycle if possible. Medical advice is needed if the patient is symptomatic.
Write the patient's name and date of birth on the opaque end of the glass slide.	For identification and correlation with the form.
Ensure the room is warm, privacy is guaranteed, and the patient has emptied her bladder.	To help the patient to relax and be comfortable during the procedure.
Ask the patient to remove the necessary clothing and lie on the couch.	To allow a clear view of the genital area.

Warm the speculum to body temperature in warm water.	To avoid discomfort for the patient.
Position the patient with her knees raised and apart, or in left lateral position. Adjust the light.	To ensure a good view of the vulva and cervix can be obtained.
Put on gloves.	For protection from possible infection.
Observe the vulva for any skin lesions, bleeding, discharge or soreness.	To detect any abnormalities or signs of infection or disease.
Remove excess water from the speculum and insert it sideways halfway into the vagina.	Water can macerate the cells. Excess lubricant can affect the quality of the cell sample.
Turn the speculum, gently manoeuvre it and open the blades.	To bring the cervix into view.
Gentle examination may be necessary if the cervix is difficult to visualise. The patient may need to lie flat with a cushion under the buttocks, if not in left lateral position.	To locate the position of the cervix manually. If the cervix is very posterior.
Vaginismus should alert the nurse to possible sexual difficulties which the patient may be encountering.	Involuntary contraction of vaginal wall muscles prevents penetration of the vagina.
Note the vaginal walls while inserting the speculum and observe the condition of the cervix.	For any problems e.g. prolapse, warts, discharge or abnormal appearance of the cervix.
Pass the tip of the spatula through the speculum and with the longest part resting in the cervical os turn the spatula through a full circle twice, using pencil-writing pressure.	To obtain cells from the transformation zone – the junction of squamous and columnar cells where pre-malignant changes are most likely to be found (Fig. 6.2).
If the cervix is eroded widen the circle of turn. Use a cervical brush if the squamo-columnar junction is not visible. (If taught to use a brush.)	The position of the squamo-columnar junction varies with age. (Fig. 6.3).
Spread the sample onto the glass slide with two long strokes – one for each side of the spatula, covering half the length of the slide each time (roll the brush, if used, along the whole slide).	To obtain a satisfactory cell sample and avoid damaging the cells. A second slide must be used for a brush.
Flood the slide with fixative, holding the bottle with a tissue.	To preserve the cells on the slide without contaminating the fixative bottle.

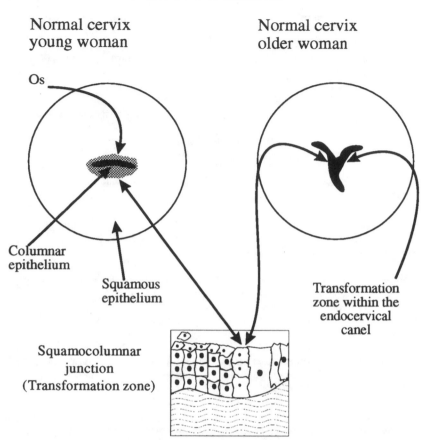

Normal cervix young woman

Normal cervix older woman

Os

Columnar epithelium

Squamous epithelium

Transformation zone within the endocervical canel

Squamocolumnar junction (Transformation zone)

Fig. 6.2   Identifying the squamo-columnar junction.

Remove the speculum and dispose of it safely.	To prevent cross-infection.
Invite the patient to get dressed if a pelvic examination is not planned.	Pelvic examination requires special training, and may not be necessary if the patient is asymptomatic[5].
Record clinical findings or technical problems on the pathology form.	To aid the cytologist's interpretation.
Allow the slide to dry then place in slide box.	For the safe transport of a well-fixed slide.

Make sure the patient knows how she will be notified of the result, and reassure her that a result asking her to consult her doctor, is as likely to indicate a technical problem as any changes in the cervical cells.

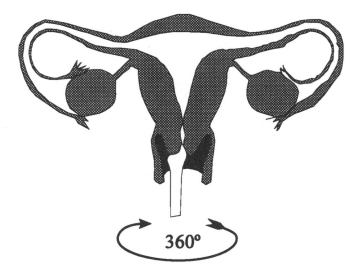

Fig. 6.3 The Aylesbury spatula in use.

Swabs

Samples of infected material can be obtained from any accessible part of the body by using a sterile swab stick tipped with cotton wool. Commercially produced swab sticks are packaged with a plastic tube containing transport medium. Once the patient has understood and agreed to the procedure, the swab should be gently rotated in the material for culture and transferred immediately to the container.

Nasal swabs

Moisten the swab with sterile saline solution because the mucosa is dry. Organisms will adhere more easily to a moist swab. Rotate the tip of the swab inside the anterior nares.

Throat swabs

A good light is required to visualise the throat. A tongue depressor may be needed to see the throat and prevent contamination of the sample if swabbing stimulates the gag reflex. Take the swab from the tonsillar area or any exudate.

Ear swabs

Rotate the swab tip gently at the entrance of the auditory meatus before any treatment drops are used. This will prevent infecting organisms being masked by the treatment drops.

Vaginal swabs

Gently part the labia to visualise the introitus and swab inside the vagina.

High vaginal swabs

Pass a speculum (as described for taking cervical smears) to visualise the cervix. Swab the discharge in the posterior fornix and withdraw the swab carefully, avoiding contact with the vaginal walls and vulva; and/or use a chlamydia swab to test for chlamydia in the endocervix.

Urethral swabs

Retract the prepuce of an uncircumcised male patient, or part the labia if a female. Swab the urethral orifice.

Rectal swabs

Gently pass the tip of the swab through the anus into the rectum. Rotate the swab and withdraw it.

Threadworms

Threadworms lay their eggs outside the anus at night. Swab the perianal area to detect threadworm ova. Alternatively instruct the patient/parent to tape a piece of cellotape next to the anus at bedtime, to collect a sample of threadworms as they emerge. Seal the tape onto a ground glass slide for microscopy.

Faeces

Specimens of faeces are usually collected by the patient at home, in a special container with a spoon attached. Instruct the patient to empty his/her bladder and then place about six layers of toilet paper into the toilet pan, pass the stool onto the paper and scoop a small section of the stool into the container with the spoon provided. The importance of hand washing should be stressed. Samples for microbiology must be taken directly to the laboratory.

Practice nurses can provide information to all patients with diarrhoea on basic hygiene and food handling. Professional food handlers with gastro-intestinal infections must have three normal stool results before returning to work[6].

Consult the laboratory about special instructions for stool specimens for occult blood or faecal fat.

Semen

Patients may be required to produce semen samples for infertility investigations or to check the effectiveness of vasectomy operations. The sample of ejaculate should be collected in a sterile wide specimen container and taken to the laboratory immediately.

Sputum

Sputum specimens can be requested for microbiology or cytology. The patient should be given a wide sterile specimen container and asked to produce a specimen of sputum after some deep productive coughing; preferably in the morning before eating or drinking. The physiotherapist may be asked to help patients who are unable to expectorate.

Investigations and tests within the practice

Blood tests

Tests performed on-site allow the results to be available more quickly.

Blood glucose

Commercially produced test strips and meters give accurate results providing a few simple rules are followed:

- Always follow the manufacturers' instructions.
- Check with the laboratory about quality control.
- Keep the test strips dry in sealed containers.
- Discard out-of-date strips.
- Use a drop of blood large enough to cover the test area.
- Use accurate timing.
- If required – wipe blood off smoothly. Do not blot it.
- Make sure the meter is calibrated to match the strips.
- Keep the meter clean and renew the battery when necessary.
- Record results immediately.

Special lancets are available on prescription. An automatic device makes the finger prick less painful by controlling the depth and speed of the puncture. A new lancet must be used for each patient. Prick the sides of the fingers rather than the tips; that way less damage is caused to sensory nerve endings[7].

Erythrocyte sedimentation rate (ESR)

ESR is a measure of how fast the red cells collect as a sediment in a vertical tube. It is a non-specific test to indicate the presence or absence of inflammatory processes. Blood can be sent to the laboratory, or the test may be performed in the surgery, using either a disposable plastic calibrated tube, or a vacuum system glass tube in a special stand.

The test should be set up according to the manufacturer's instructions and the level of sedimentation noted after one hour. An automatic timer can help to ensure a reading is not forgotten. After an hour the sedimentation rate becomes more rapid, so can give a falsely high reading.

The normal ESR range is 3–10mm/hr for men and 5–15mm/hr for women although measurements just above the range are common and need to be interpreted carefully.

Clinical chemistry analysis

Compact microprocessor instruments are already available for performing a range of blood and urine tests on-site. Results can be printed out for the patients' records. As yet, the systems are costly and do not have any significant advantages over laboratory services[8]. In the future, advances in the technology and price reductions, could lead to many more tests being carried out in the practice.

Urine tests

A range of diptests are available for urinalysis. They have a limited shelf life once opened and some are very costly. It pays to select the most suitable product for the tests required (see Fig. 6.4). Multistix 8SG are now available in smaller quantities, more suitable for use in general practice. All test strips must be kept dry, with the bottle top replaced immediately after use. The desiccant sachet must not be removed. The type of test should be specified when recording results. Urine specimens should be emptied into a toilet rather than a sink.

Pregnancy tests

Easy-to-use pregnancy tests such as *Clearview* can be purchased in

SOME EXAMPLES OF URINE DIPTESTS	
Substance	**Product**
Single tests	
Protein	Albustix[*]
Glucose	Diastix[*]
Ketones	Ketostix[*]
Combinations	
Protein & glucose	Uristix
Glucose & ketones	Keto-diastix
pH, protein, glucose ketones, blood & nitrite	N-Labstix
pH, protein, glucose ketones, blood & bilirubin	Bili-Labsix
pH, protein, glucose ketones, specific gravity blood, nitrite & leucocytes	Multistix 8SG
pH, protein, glucose, ketones specific gravity, blood nitrite, leucocytes, bilirubin and urobilinogen	Multistix 10SG

[*] Available on FP10 prescription.

Fig. 6.4 Examples of urine diptests.

bulk. Five drops of urine are dropped onto the test pad. If a blue line appears in the middle panel after two minutes the test is positive. A blue line should show in the top panel, whatever the result, as a quality control.

The tests are expensive and cannot be reimbursed, so a policy is needed about when they should be performed. If a patient has done a positive home test, there is little point in repeating it. Patients who request tests too frequently may have other concerns about contraception, and need help or advice.

Microscopy

The use of a microscope is mainly limited to looking for pus cells in urine when a urinary tract infection is suspected. Although other uses include looking for fungal hyphae in nail or skin scrapings, trichomonas vaginalis in vaginal discharge, or for looking at blood smears. The degree of microscope use might depend on the accessibility of a pathology laboratory but it can provide the opportunity to commence treatment before laboratory results are available.

Arrangements can be made in-house, or through the laboratory, for practice nurses to learn how to prepare slides and use the microscope.

Respiratory function tests

Peak expiratory flow rate (PEFR)

Peak flow meters measure the amount of air which a patient is capable of expelling forcibly from the lungs. It is not the volume of air which is measured, but the rate of expulsion. This is directly related to the elasticity of the lungs and the volume of air within the lungs, and is measured in litres per minute expelled. The normal range for an adult male of about 1.80m in height would be 550–700 l/min. The normal varies according to height, sex and age. Tables are provided with each instrument to give guidance on this. These guides constitute the 'predicted' levels against which an individual patient's results can be compared.

Use of a peak flow meter is vital to the modern treatment of asthma. Indeed many patients with asthma are encouraged to keep one at home and use it regularly. A fall in the peak flow rate may be the first indication of the onset of severe asthma. (See Chapter 7, *Emergency Situations* and Chapter 15, *Asthma*).

The modern equivalent of the Wright's peak flow meter – the Mini-Wright's meter, is a small plastic tube with a scale along the top and a movable indicator. This type, and similar meters, can be prescribed on FP10. The readings from different types of peak flow meters are not always comparable[9].

In the surgery a peak flow meter may be used in health screening for smokers, as well as patients with a history of airways disease.

Action	Rationale
Ask the patient to stand up.	To allow the maximum expansion of the chest.
Explain the procedure.	To ensure compliance.
Ask the patient to hold the meter horizontally and to keep the fingers away from the cursor.	To allow the cursor to move freely along the scale.
Then to take a slow deep breath, place the lips around the mouthpiece and to breathe out as quickly and forcibly as possible.	To expand the lungs fully. To expel the air from the lungs.

If the procedure has been performed correctly, or the patient is not too breathless, the cursor will move along the scale and the reading can be taken. The whole manoeuvre can then be repeated two more times, and the best of the three readings recorded and compared with the predicted level for the patient's age and height.

Spirometry

Some practices now own micro spirometers for recording the forced expiratory volume, the amount that can be breathed out in one second (FEV_1) and the forced vital capacity – the total amount exhaled after a maximum inhalation. The manufacturer's instructions for the use of the instrument should be followed. The procedure is similar to peak flow recording except that the patient is asked to blow into the mouthpiece as hard and fast and as *long* as possible. The results can be read from the liquid crystal display and compared with predicted levels.

Electrocardiography

The ECG records electrical potential in the heart muscle as it beats. The various electrical pathways are altered in muscle which has been damaged or where the heart is beating irregularly. These changes give the tracing its characteristic appearance and assist in the diagnosis of cardiac problems. Occasionally a patient may be asked to exercise under supervision before the recording is made.

Machines vary, so the maker's instruction must be followed. Nurses who have not worked in coronary care require training in the recording and interpretation of ECGs.

Requirements

ECG machine with disposable or reusable electrodes
Contact jelly/cream
Ball-point pen
Tissues

Action	Rationale
Ensure privacy and a warm room temperature.	The patient will need to undress and shivering will affect the tracing.
Make sure the patient knows what to expect and that it will be painless.	The wires and straps can look like something from a horror movie and cause unnecessary anxiety.
Ask the patient to undress as needed, assist him/her onto the couch and make as comfortable as possible.	The chest, wrists and ankles will need to be accessible. So he/she can lie still during the procedure.
Smear the electrodes with some contact jelly and attach them to the wrists and ankles with the straps (if not using adhesive electrodes).	To create a good contact between the skin and the electrodes.
Chest leads may be attached at the same time, or later.	Depending on the type of ECG machine being used. (Fig. 6.5.)
Attach the correct wires to the electrodes.	To allow the machine to pick up the electrical impulses.
Begin the tracing when the patient is relaxed.	Movement will cause electrical interference.
Calibrate the tracing by pressing the appropriate button on the machine.	To allow the reader to assess the size of the various wavelengths.
Record leads I, II, III, aVR, aVL and aVF in turn.	To record electrical potential from different directions.
Record approximately five complexes per tracing.	To allow an adequate reading without wasting recording paper.
Record a longer tracing of II (10–12 complexes).	To act as a rhythm strip. Lead II is usually closest to the cardiac vector. (The direction and strength of electrical voltage of the heart as it contracts.)
Mark the tracings with a ball-point pen.	To help the reader identify each tracing and compare it with the norm.

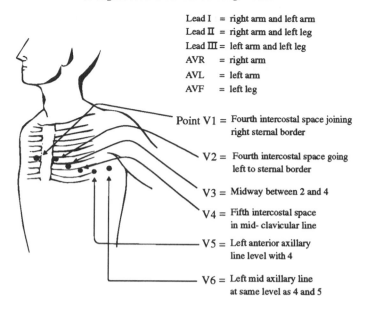

Lead I   = right arm and left arm
Lead II = right arm and left leg
Lead III = left arm and left leg
AVR   = right arm
AVL   = left arm
AVF   = left leg

Point V1 = Fourth intercostal space joining right sternal border

V2 = Fourth intercostal space going left to sternal border

V3 = Midway between 2 and 4

V4 = Fifth intercostal space in mid- clavicular line

V5 = Left anterior axillary line level with 4

V6 = Left mid axillary line at same level as 4 and 5

Fig. 6.5   Siting the ECG chest leads.

Attach the chest leads using a suction cup and contact jelly if adhesive electrodes are not available.

To pick up the electrical impulses from different areas around the heart.

Turn the machine to V setting (if a manual machine). Record the six V tracings (Fig. 6.5).

Problems which may occur

Machine not recording:

- check that the plugs are pushed in properly and the electricity is switched on,
- check that the machine has not run out of paper.

Interference with the ECG tracing:

- There may be interfence from other electrical equipment or the metal frame of the couch.
- Check the electrodes are giving good skin contact. (Hairy chests and arms may need to be shaved.)

- Check the wires are attached to the correct electrodes.
- The machine may need servicing.

When all the tracings have been taken satisfactorily remove the electrodes, wipe the contact jelly/cream off the skin and invite the patient to get dressed.

Interpreting results

Nurses who perform electrocardiography must be able to recognise a normal and abnormal tracing so that medical advice can be obtained if needed before the patient leaves the surgery. The protocol should cover the action to be taken in event of an abnormal tracing. A few examples of common conditions are shown in Fig. 6.6.

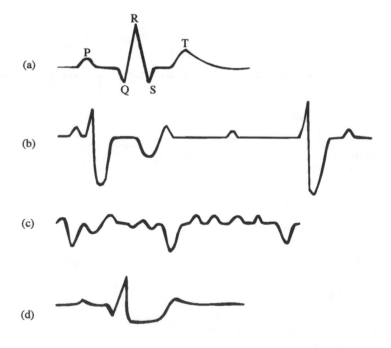

Fig. 6.6 Examples of ECG tracings. (a) Basic recording. (b) Complete heart block (conduction defect). (c) Atrial fibrillation. (d) ST depression in myocardial infarction.

Screening audiometry

Hearing tests for young children are undertaken by health visitors, or at hearing clinics. Other patients suspected of hearing loss may be referred to the practice nurse for a screening audiogram. This procedure will usually indicate in adults, and children old enough to participate, a hearing problem which requires further investigation. A history should be noted of any ear infections or injuries, speech or learning difficulties, or family history of deafness.

A screening audiogram entails recording the quietest sound the patient can hear in a range of frequencies (usually 500, 1000 and 4000 Hz), working down in 5–10 decibel steps from 60 or 30 dB. A quiet room is needed for the test. Distractions must be avoided as concentration may be lost. Children can be encouraged to participate in the test by playing a game. For example – a marble put into a jar every time a sound is heard.

The machine must be checked before use, be serviced and re-calibrated annually. A record should be kept of the service date.

Action	Rationale
Examine the ears.	For wax, signs of infection or congestion.
Postpone the test if necessary.	If treatment is required for wax or infection.
Explain the test procedure.	To gain co-operation and allay any fears.
Arrange the way the patient will indicate when a sound is heard. Make a game for children.	The machine may have a button to depress, or he/she may raise a hand. (See above).
Position the headphones comfortably.	To ensure extraneous noise is excluded.
Place the test machine where the patient does not see it.	So the patient is not influenced by seeing the buttons being depressed.
Start with a middle frequency (1000 Hz).	Higher and lower sounds are more likely to be lost.
Begin at about 30 dB and if the patient responds, reduce in 10 dB steps until the patient no longer responds. Make each sound for approximately three seconds.	To establish the smallest sound the patient can hear.
Use a higher volume if necessary.	If the patient does not hear 30 or 40 dB.
Try 5 dB above and below the lowest sound heard.	To be sure of the exact point.

Record the level on the graph. Mark X for the left ear, and O for the right.

The hearing of both ears can be compared (Fig. 6.7).

Repeat the procedure at a high frequency (4000 Hz) and low frequency (500 Hz).

Hearing may not be lost uniformly.

Other frequencies may also be recorded, depending on the equipment and practice policy. Children will get bored if the test is prolonged. If it is unclear whether a patient, particularly a child, is responding appropriately, the audiometer can be turned off. It will soon become apparent if the patient responds when no sounds are being made.

If there is obvious hearing loss, or a dubious result, the patient should be referred for specialised hearing tests in an ENT department. Some patients will benefit from using a hearing aid. It is better to learn to use them while young enough to adapt. Practice nurses can encourage patients to persevere with their aids, to prevent social isolation in old age.

Visual acuity test

Visual acuity is tested by reading letters of decreasing size at a measured distance from a Snellen chart. Special charts are available for patients who are illiterate or too young to read. The Snellen chart should be attached to the wall and be well-illuminated. A patient who normally

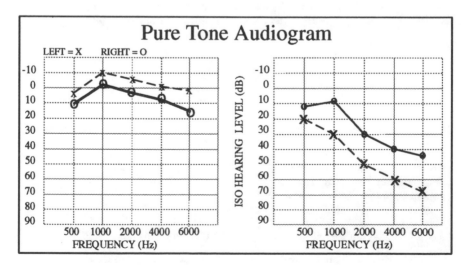

Fig. 6.7 Examples of audiogram recordings.

wears spectacles for distance vision should be tested with the glasses on with this noted on the record.

Action	Rationale
Measure six metres from the chart.	The chart is designed to be read at this distance.
Position the patient at the six metre mark.	
Ask the patient to cover one eye gently.	Each eye is tested in turn.
Ask the patient to read the letters on the chart starting from the top.	To discover the smallest letters which can be read correctly.
Record the number of the last complete line to be read accurately.	Each line is marked with the distance at which it can be read by a normal eye.
Repeat the procedure with the other eye.	

The largest letter can be read by a person with normal sight from 60 metres, and the smallest letters from four metres. The result of a person reading from six metres distance who can read the sixth line (9m) is written as 6/9. The test result of a patient with poor vision who can only see the top line is written as 6/60.

Patients who cannot see any of the letters on the chart may be tested to see if they can identify hand movements, or are able to perceive light.

Suggestions for evaluation and research

- Review the practice procedure for dealing with test results. Is there any way that abnormal results could be overlooked?
- Devise a study of urine diptests. Are the most appropriate products being used for the type of tests required?
- Conduct a literature search on the advantages and disadvantages of using peak flow meters.

References

1. News (1993) Smear case highlights lack of training; *Community Outlook*, October: 9.
2. World Health Organisation (1990) *Guidelines for Counselling People with HIV.* WHO, Geneva.

3. Royal Mail (1993) *Prohibited and Restricted Goods: a Few Limitations on Goods which can be sent by Post*. Booklet available from Royal Mail Customer Service Centres.
4. Tietz, N. (Ed.) (1983) *Clinical Guide to Laboratory Tests*: 92–93. Saunders.
5. Austoker, J. (1993) Routine bi-manual pelvic examination. Annual conference report in the *RCN Family Planning Forum Winter Newsletter*. RCN, London.
6. Great Britain, Parliament (1984) *Public Health (Control of Disease) Act 1984*. HMSO, London.
7. Steward, E. (1990) Blood glucose monitoring (Fig 2b, c); *Practice Nurse*, **2**: 368.
8. Rink, E., Hilton, S., Szczepure, A., Fletcher, J., Sibbald, B., Davies, C., Freeling, P. and Stilwell, J. (1993) Impact of introducing near patient testing for standard investigations in general practice; *British Medical Journal*, **307**: 775–778.
9. Miller, M.R., Dickinson, S.A. and Hitchings, D.J. (1991) Accuracy of measurements of peak flow with different peak flow meters; *Thorax*, **46**: 289.

Further reading

Thorpe, S. (1991) *A Practical Guide to Taking Blood*. Bailliere Tindall, London.
Ames (1990) *Urinalysis, the Inside Information*. Bayer Diagnostics, Basingstoke.
Royal College of Nursing (1991) *Family Planning Manual for Nurses*. Scutari, Harrow.
Inglis, T. and West, A. (1993) *Colour Guide to Microbiology*. Churchill Livingstone, Edinburgh.

Chapter 7
Emergency Situations

From time-to-time life-threatening crises will occur in the practice. In addition, a practice nurse will sometimes be the only professionally qualified member of staff on the premises when an emergency call is received. She/he will be expected to assess the degree of urgency of the request and to assist the reception staff in deciding on the appropriate course of action to take.

Accidents by their very nature happen without warning, but many of them could be anticipated and prevented. The objective of one of the five key areas in the *Health of the Nation* white paper is a reduction in ill-health, disability and death caused by accidents or unintentional injuries[1]. So apart from dealing with any emergencies which occur, medical and nursing staff also have a role in educating patients about safety. Information should be available in the surgery about road safety and the prevention of accidents in the home and workplace.

General principles

The basic principles of first aid should always be kept in mind in the event of an emergency. M. Skeet states that first aid is given to:

- sustain life
- prevent the condition from becoming worse
- promote recovery[2].

While a practice nurse is unlikely to encounter situations involving multiple casualties, nevertheless she/he must always be aware that these could happen, and first aid skills need to be kept up-to-date. The following general principles always apply:

Action	Rationale
Check that it is safe to approach the patient.	To avoid putting yourself and others at risk.
Maintain a calm manner and take charge confidently.	To prevent panic and to resist the pressure to act in haste.
Collect as much relevant information as possible.	To assess the situation and decide on the priorities for action.
Deal with life-threatening emergencies immediately.	To maintain the patient's respiration and circulation.
Arrange for medical help from the GP, or ambulance service.	This depends on the perceived severity of the problem.

Practice nurses will often be able to deal with minor trauma themselves. Whether giving advice over the telephone, rendering first aid at the site of an accident, or dealing with an incident in the surgery, three factors require priority:

- **A – Airway**   – must be clear for air entry to the lungs,
- **B – Breathing**   – must be present to oxygenate the blood,
- **C – Circulation** – is essential for perfusion of the brain and vital organs[3].

Asphyxia

Blockage of the airway, so that the brain is starved of oxygen, can occur in ways ranging from inhalation of a foreign body, to crush injuries in an accident. The principles for treatment do not differ. Suction apparatus should be available in the treatment room, together with airways in a range of sizes and adult and paediatric resuscitation masks. Oxygen can also be needed at times.

Diagnosis

The history may make this obvious (e.g. the mother sees a child swallow a marble and the child then goes blue and chokes). However, in other situations such as an unconscious patient, the cause may not be known.

A patient who collapses at the dining table may have choked on a piece of food, but be diagnosed mistakenly as having had a heart attack. Any patient who collapses while eating should be assumed to have choked until proved otherwise.

An asphyxiated patient loses consciousness quickly and the face and extremities become cyanosed. Death will follow if prompt action is not taken. If asphyxia is due to an inhaled foreign body then several manoeuvres may help.

Infants

- Position the baby head-down along your forearm and support the chin with your hand, to make use of gravity to dislodge the obstruction and to maintain the clear airway position.
- Tap between the baby's shoulder-blades up to five times with appropriate force, to try to dislodge the foreign body.
- Check for breathing in case artificial respiration is necessary (see *Collapse* below).
- Repeat the procedure or treat as an unconscious patient, as the situation warrants.

Children

Sit with the child head-down over your knee and continue the procedure as for a baby. Use slightly more force for the back blows.

Adults

Bend the patient forward with the head lower than the chest. Give five sharp slaps with the heel of your hand. If the obstruction is not cleared, try abdominal thrusts. Stand behind the patient, clasp your hands below his/her xiphisternum. Pull sharply upwards and inwards under the patient's sternum. Air is forced up the airway by the sudden pressure under the diaphragm and hopefully will expel the obstruction (Fig. 7.1 Heimlich manoeuvre).

Repeat four more times if the first manoeuvres fail, and alternate with back blows. If the patient loses consciousness check the breathing. The muscles may relax after consciousness is lost. If the airway is not clear – try five back blows and follow with up to five abdominal thrusts. Kneel astride the patient and press inwards and upwards under the diaphragm, using the heel of one hand with the other on top of it. Follow the *collapse* procedure.

Collapse

Any sudden prostration or loss of consciousness is loosely termed 'collapse'. The reason may be obvious when it happens in the surgery, but on other occasions an assessment of all the clues will be needed.

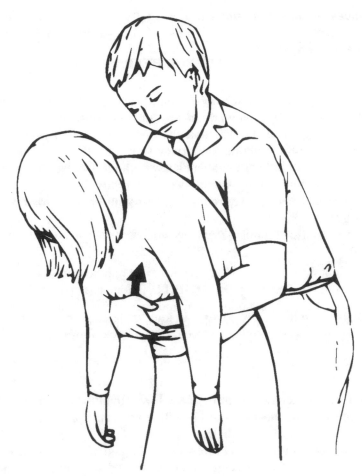

Fig. 7.1   Heimlich manoeuvre.

Four courses of action are possible, whatever the cause of the collapse[4].

Collapsed but conscious patient

(1)   Check it is safe to approach.
(2)   Attempt to rouse the patient. Does the patient respond to calling or a gentle shake of the shoulders?
      If yes – obtain information about his/her condition, treat as appropriate and call for help if needed.

Collapsed unconscious patient

Check **1** and **2** as above.

 If there is no response – **CALL FOR HELP**.

A – Check that the upper airway is clear. Leave well-fitting dentures in place but clear the mouth of any obvious obstruction. Tilt the patient's head backwards and lift the lower jaw to prevent the tongue from obstructing the airway (Fig. 7.2). If a spinal injury is suspected try lifting the patient's jaw without moving the head.

B – Check the patient is breathing – watch the chest, listen for breathing sounds and feel for expired air against your cheek – for five seconds.

C – Check the carotid pulse for five seconds.

If the patient is breathing and has a pulse turn him/her into the recovery position (see Fig. 7.3) and **GO FOR HELP**, if none has arrived. Re-check the pulse and breathing upon return and regularly until help arrives.

 Control any haemorrhage or life-threatening injury.

Respiratory arrest

Check **1** and **2**. If no response – **CALL FOR HELP**.

 Check **ABC** (see above).

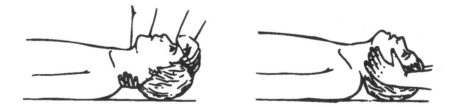

Fig. 7.2 Extension of the patient's neck to maintain the airway.

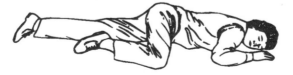

Fig. 7.3 Recovery or coma position.

If the patient has a clear airway and pulse present but is not breathing start mouth-to-mouth, or mouth-to-mask resuscitation.

Open the airway, close the nostrils and give ten slow breaths with a 2–4 second pause between each. Watch to see the chest fall after each inflation. After ten breaths check for breathing and pulse. If no assistance has arrived place the patient in the recovery position and **GO FOR HELP**. (Telephone for an ambulance.)

Check the breathing and pulse on your return. If a pulse is present but still no breathing, continue artificial ventilation until help arrives. Check for breathing and pulse after every ten breaths. If the patient starts breathing spontaneously place him/her in the recovery position and continue to observe.

Cardiac arrest

Check **1** and **2** (see above).

  If no response – **CALL FOR HELP**.

  Check **ABC** (see above).

Clear the mouth if necessary and position the head and jaw to open the airway. If not breathing and no pulse – **GO FOR HELP**, if none has arrived. (Telephone for an ambulance.)

Quickly reassess when you return. Start cardio-pulmonary resuscitation (CPR) if the pulse and breathing are still absent.

One person resuscitation (adults)

Give two slow breaths then 15 chest compressions. Kneel beside the patient's chest. Place the heel of one hand two fingers' width above the xiphisternum, place your other hand over the first and lock the fingers, to avoid pressure on the patient's ribs. Keep your arms straight, lean forward, and use your body weight to compress the sternum (4–5cm). Repeat the sequence until help arrives.

Two person resuscitation (adults)

Give one slow breath to every five compressions. The person performing the compressions should count the rhythm.

DO NOT STOP THE BASIC LIFE SUPPORT TO CHECK FOR A PULSE (unless the patient moves). Keep going until the ambulance arrives.

There are several differences in the technique for resuscitating infants and children. Every district has a training officer and all doctors and nurses are advised to undertake regular training in resuscitation, because these skills are easily lost when they are needed so rarely.

Common emergencies in practice and first aid management

Fainting (vasovagal syncope)

Probably the commonest cause of collapse in the treatment room is a faint. Most patients get some warning of this. They become very pale and sweaty and feel nauseated, and they may lose consciousness. The pulse will be slow.

If a patient who feels faint lies flat or sits with the head lowered between the knees, this will often prevent the faint from occurring. (Warning – a very pregnant woman should lie on her side because the enlarged uterus can press on the inferior vena cava and compound the problem by slowing the venous return.)

A patient who has collapsed from a simple faint will quickly recover when horizontal and this can be a useful diagnostic pointer to the cause of the collapse.

Anaphylaxis

Anaphylactic shock is a life-threatening condition caused by an acute allergic reaction to an injected drug or insect sting. Ingested food or medicines can also cause severe reactions, usually of slower onset. The allergen causes histamine and other powerful substances to be released, which then cause:

- urticaria
- peripheral vasodilatation and oedema
- laryngeal stridor
- bronchospasm and tachycardia.

Characteristically the patient has a sense of impending death. The blood pressure falls and vital organs are starved of oxygen. The action to be taken in such an event must be established in advance, with a protocol and emergency drugs always available. Request medical assistance once anaphylaxis has been diagnosed, but initiate the treatment immediately:

Action	Rationale
Support the patient in the most comfortable position.	To assist breathing if dyspnoeic or restless.
Or: Place in the recovery position if unconscious and insert an oral airway.	To protect the airway from being obstructed.
Administer adrenaline in the appropriate dose I/M (see Fig. 7.4).	To constrict the peripheral blood vessels to raise the blood pressure.
Monitor the BP and respiration. Repeat adrenaline after 10 min.	To assess the response to the treatment. If there is no improvement.
Begin CPR if appropriate.	To maintain the blood and O_2 supply to the vital centres.
IV hydrocortisone 100mg may be given by the GP.	For its anti-inflammatory effect.
Transfer the patient to hospital.	Delayed reactions can still occur.

If anaphylaxis occurs after an injection, save the syringe and vial if possible, in case they are needed for examination.

Age	Dose
< 6 months	0.05ml
6-11 months	0.075ml
1 year	0.1ml
2 years	0.2ml
3-4 years	0.3ml
5 years and over	0.5ml
Adults	0.5-1ml

Fig. 7.4 Adrenaline doses according to age.

Myocardial infarction

Patients with severe angina or a frank myocardial infarct will sometimes arrive in surgery unaware how ill they are. The classical symptoms are severe, crushing, central chest pain with or without radiation to the jaw and left arm. The patient may feel very unwell, and look pale and sweaty. However these gross symptoms are not always present and a patient may collapse without warning. In either case, assess the situation and call for an ambulance if no doctor is on the premises. If the patient is conscious obtain as much information as possible to help make the diagnosis. Sit the patient in the most comfortable position to assist his/her breathing and if the patient carries trinitrin or similar medication administer a dose to increase the cardiac perfusion[5]. Give one aspirin for its anti-thrombotic effect if MI is suspected, but enquire about salicylate allergy first. Check the pulse and blood pressure to monitor progress and identify a deteriorating condition.

If cardiac arrest occurs follow the procedure set out above (see *Collapse*).

If an emergency call is received when no doctor is immediately available for a patient who has collapsed at home with symptoms suggestive of a myocardial infarction, then it is best to summon the help of ambulance personnel and continue trying to contact the doctor.

Transient ischaemic attacks

Atherosclerosis may affect the whole arterial tree in some older patients. From time-to-time this may result in the normal physiological mechanisms for maintaining the blood flow to be slightly delayed; the cerebral circulation is particularly sensitive in this situation. A sudden change in posture, turning the head quickly or other quick movement may cause the patient to be transiently giddy or even faint, but recovery is almost instantaneous. Patients can usually be reassured and advised to try and change position more slowly.

Collections of platelets over atheromatous plaques can break off, lodge as emboli in the cerebral circulation and cause mild stroke symptoms. Recovery can take about 24 hours as the emboli disperse, but the process is likely to be frightening for the patient and carers. A medical examination will be necessary in most instances.

Cerebrovascular episode (stroke, CVA)

A cerebral thrombosis, embolus or haemorrhage can cause a more major cerebral catastrophe resulting in unconsciousness, hemiparesis or hemiplegia. The action to take if it occurs in the surgery is that for a collapsed patient. If it occurs at home, the relatives should be advised to make the patient as comfortable as possible wherever he/she has fallen, to maintain a clear airway, and to turn the patient into the recovery position if unconscious. The decision about admission to hospital should be made after all the circumstances have been considered, but it will often be possible to wait until the doctor has seen the patient.

Convulsions

Epileptic seizures

A generalised seizure can be frightening both for the patient and any onlookers. A practice nurse's role can involve more than simply helping a patient who has a seizure in the surgery. Some nurses are using their expertise to give longer-term support to patients with epilepsy and their families (see Chapter 15). In the event of a tonic-clonic seizure in the surgery the principles are straightforward:

Action	Rationale
Give the patient as much room as possible and try to ease the fall.	To prevent injury from hitting furniture or sharp corners.
Protect the head with a pillow if possible.	To prevent unnecessary trauma.
Do not attempt to wedge anything into the mouth.	More damage is likely to be caused and there is a danger of being bitten.
Note the time and sequence of events.	To aid the diagnosis, especially if a first fit.
Put the patient in the recovery position once the seizure is over.	To protect the airway until consciousness is regained.

Once consciousness has been regained and the patient is talking coherently he/she can go home with a friend or relative, after verifying some details. The nurse must check whether the patient is taking medication regularly and has an adequate supply. An urgent medical examination is needed after a fit by any patient who is not known to have epilepsy.

Transfer to hospital should be arranged if repeated or uncontrolled seizures occur, or the patient does not regain consciousness after ten minutes[6].

Febrile convulsions

Babies and young children may develop convulsions in response to a febrile illness. A child will usually look hot, flushed and obviously feverish, with violent unco-ordinated movements. Also he/she may be cyanosed from breath-holding, have twitching of the face and rolled up eyes.

Action	Rationale
Remove the child's clothing and sponge the skin with tepid water.	To cool the skin by evaporation and so lower the body temperature.
Position the child on something soft.	To prevent injury during convulsive movements.
Meanwhile, explain to the parents what is happening.	They are bound to be very anxious if they have never seen a febrile convulsion.
Arrange for the child to be transferred to hospital if no doctor is immediately available.	To identify and treat the cause of the fever, and to reassure the parents.

Head injury

A very young child and any patient who has been unconscious after a head injury, must be examined by a doctor. However, a practice nurse may sometimes see an active, alert child whose mother wants reassurance after the child sustained a fall or blow to the head. The assessment of a head injury should:

- Establish the circumstances of the injury.
- Ensure there was no loss of consciousness, or any other injuries.
- Ask if the patient remembers what happened.
- Ask if the patient has felt dizzy, nauseated or has vomited.
- Check for signs of cerebral compression.
- Check for CSF leaking from the nose or ears.

Cerebral compression may occur at the time of injury as a result of trauma to the brain, but can also develop some time after a head injury if a subdural haematoma forms. Clear instructions about what signs to look for must be given before a patient goes home. Mild headaches, dizziness or irritability are not unusual after a head injury[7]. If the symptoms persist or get worse; or if severe vomiting, limb weakness, severe drowsiness, increasing irritability or photophobia develop, the GP must be informed.

Hypoglycaemia

Diabetic patients on insulin are always at risk of having a hypoglycaemic attack and should be aware of this. Part of their education about diabetes is to explain the risks of hypoglycaemia and each patient should know the early signs so that action can be taken before unconsciousness supervenes.

The first sign of an impending hypoglycaemic attack is usually a feeling of faintness and hunger. This quickly passes on to confusion, aggressive behaviour and finally coma. The patient is pale, sweating and restless. Occasionally convulsions may occur, which can be mistaken for epilepsy. The hypoglycaemic coma is a true emergency because the longer the patient is unconscious, the greater the risk of permanent brain damage from the low blood sugar. Thus the aim of immediate treatment is to raise the blood sugar to a normal level.

- If the patient is conscious give approximately 10g of easily digested carbohydrate, e.g.: two teaspoons of sugar or glucose, three glucose tablets, or 100ml Lucozade. Follow up with 10–20g of complex carbohydrate once the patient has recovered, e.g.: 1–2 digestive biscuits, 150–300ml of milk. Alternatively the patient should be advised to have a snack or meal if it is due.
- If the patient is unresponsive, Hypostop dextrose gel in a tube can be squeezed inside the patient's cheek, to be absorbed through the buccal mucosa.
- Intramuscular Glucagon can be given to an unconscious patient, followed by 30g carbohydrate once consciousness is regained.
- The GP may need to give intravenous dextrose if all else fails.

The patient should be reviewed after a hypoglycaemic incident, to try and identify the cause and see if adjustments are needed to the treatment, diet, or lifestyle[8]. Patients who are prone to hypoglycaemia should wear or carry something to identify them as diabetic, e.g. Medic Alert bracelets or medallions.

Respiratory problems

Hyperventilation

Overbreathing can be associated with anxiety or emotional distress. Rapid deep breathing can cause faintness, trembling and carpo-pedal spasm as the carbon dioxide is breathed out and the acid/base balance is disturbed. The symptoms can cause further anxiety and so exacerbate the problem. A firm but quiet manner should be adopted. Take the patient to a quiet room, to help him/her to calm down. Try to establish what has happened. Other causes of respiratory distress need to be ruled out. Rebreathing carbon dioxide in expired air will restore the pCO_2 to its correct level, so if necessary, the patient can breathe in and out of a paper bag.

Once the patient has recovered, help can be offered to try and deal with the underlying problems.

Acute asthma

There are always likely to be some patients who require emergency treatment for an acute attack of asthma, despite the general improvements in asthma management. Practice nurses should have a protocol to follow in the event of an emergency when a doctor is not present. The following should be assessed:

- Age of the patient and previous history – is the patient known to have asthma?
- Details of the present episode – duration, and treatment already taken? Are there any known trigger factors?
- Degree of distress – is the patient able to talk? Are accessory muscles being used to breathe?
- Peak expiratory flow rate – in comparison with the predicted level, if able to use a meter. (See Chapter 6.)
- Pulse and respiration rates – there may be tachycardia and rapid respirations.

Action	Rationale
Call for medical help (or an ambulance if the patient's condition warrants it).	As this is a medical emergency.
Nebulise with salbutamol 2.5mg for children, 5mg for adults.	For the immediate relief of bronchospasm.
Monitor the patient's pulse and appearance while using the nebuliser.	To detect any change or deterioration in his/her condition.
Recheck the PEFR, pulse and respiration after nebulising.	To determine the effectiveness of the treatment.

Once the bronchospasm has been relieved, the patient must see a doctor. Usually steroids are needed to deal with the inflammation of the airways. Admission to hospital may be necessary, but in any event, the patient will need a follow-up appointment (see Chapter 15, *Asthma*).

The nebuliser attachments must be cleaned and disinfected after use, before being used for another patient.

Haemorrhage

Most cuts and minor haemorrhage will soon stop if simple pressure is applied to the site of bleeding. Gloves must be worn when dealing with any bleeding because of the risk of blood-borne infections.

Arterial bleeding

The bleeding will be profuse if an injury has severed an artery. The blood will be bright red and pumping out of the wound. Local pressure is the first act, followed by elevation of the limb, where relevant. Occasionally pressure will have to be exerted over the artery supplying the wound area. For example – in the groin, compress the femoral artery against the symphysis pubis, or in the upper arm, compress the brachial artery against the humerus. In an open wound an artery can sometimes be seen to be bleeding – if so, then the direct application of an artery forceps to the cut end is the most effective way to control the bleeding. If the blood volume is reduced significantly, the patient will become shocked, with a weak rapid pulse and fall in blood pressure. Urgent transfer to hospital will be needed. Meanwhile lay the patient down and elevate his/her legs, if possible, to aid the venous return. Make sure there is no tight clothing and keep the patient warm but not overheated. Do not give anything to drink because an anaesthetic may be necessary, or vomiting may obstruct the airway if consciousness is lost.

Varicose veins

Occasionally a patient with varicose veins will knock his/her leg and puncture a vein. The bleeding is impressive but, being venous the blood is darker, slower flowing and not pumping out. The wound itself may be almost invisible but still bleed copiously. The treatment is simple – lay the patient down, put a pad on the wound, elevate the leg and wait for the bleeding to stop. After the patient has been lying down for half an hour with the leg elevated, a firm pad and bandage can be applied, and the patient may go home if medically fit. An appointment should be made for review of the wound. The management of varicose veins and the use of support stockings can then be discussed.

Haematemesis

Haematemesis is unlikely to occur in the surgery, but occasionally a call may be received. Most episodes of vomiting blood are significant but not desperately urgent, unless a large and obvious quantity has been produced, when the patient will rapidly become shocked. This call requires urgent hospital admission, but more minor cases can be reassured and rested until a doctor can assess them.

Swallowed blood from the posterior nasal space is often mistaken for haematemesis and this cause should be considered. Taking an accurate history usually clarifies the issue.

Melaena

Bleeding within the bowel can often be overlooked in a patient who collapses with no apparent cause. A more common presentation is an unexplained iron-deficiency anaemia. Non-steroidal anti-inflammatory drugs are a common cause of gastro-intestinal bleeding, especially in the elderly. Stool samples for occult blood may be requested if bleeding is suspected. The traditional black, tarry stool of the severe melaena makes recognition of the problem easy for the doctor or nurse. Patients with frank melaena require further investigations in hospital.

A doctor should examine all patients with unexplained bleeding. Bright blood may come from haemorrhoids, but the possibility of a malignancy should always be considered.

Epistaxis

Nosebleeds are very common, particularly in children. A practice nurse may have to give advice over the telephone or to deal with the situation in the surgery. A calm manner will help to reassure the patient.

- Seat the patient with his/her head forward to prevent blood from running down the back of the throat.
- Instruct the patient to pinch the fleshy part of the nose between his/her finger and thumb for a *timed* 10 minutes and to breathe through the mouth. This action should compress the bleeding point long enough to allow clotting to take place. It is not possible to guess the time accurately enough – a clock or watch must be used.

This action will stop a very high proportion of nosebleeds in children and some adults. A clot which has formed in the nostril should be left alone and not blown out as this will restart the bleeding. Recurrent nosebleeds in children are often due to a dilated single capillary in the lower part of the nasal septum and in these instances the GP may want to cauterise the vessel.

In adults, the bleeding sometimes occurs from higher up the nose and may be precipitated by the rupture of a small arteriosclerotic capillary. Hypertension must be considered as a cause of nosebleeds; so it is always worth taking the blood pressure and pulse. This can become useful information if the bleeding becomes profuse. Occasionally adults need hospital admission if the bleeding will not stop.

If the simple pressure technique does not stop the bleeding after several attempts, then the nose may need to be packed by a doctor.

Poisoning

Young children will put anything in their mouths. An anxious parent may rush to the surgery for help when an accident occurs. If the child is unconscious or known to have ingested a really hazardous substance, then call for an emergency ambulance immediately if no doctor is present. Otherwise try to calm the parent and collect as much information as possible – what was taken, how much and when?

- Do not try to induce vomiting – caustic substances may cause further damage to the oesophagus, and volatile substances may affect the lungs.
- Consult the Poisons Reference Centre – to find the correct action to take (if the substance swallowed can be identified).
- Save any vomit – in case it is needed for analysis.

This action would apply equally to adults who have been poisoned – either accidentally or through drug overdose. Abuse of alcohol, drugs and solvents can cause a patient to collapse.

Pain

Individuals have different tolerance levels for pain but a patient who attends the surgery with symptoms of pain will require a careful assessment. The nerve pathways and factors which influence the perception of pain are complex. The method of pain relief will vary with its cause, and if a nurse is required to assess a patient's pain, the following points should be considered:

- Type of pain – constant or intermittent, throbbing, burning, stabbing?
- Onset and duration – how long has the patient been in pain?
- Does anything help – position, analgesics, antacids?
- Intensity of pain – on a scale of 1–10, with 1 as very mild, to 10 as the worst pain imaginable.
- Localisation – can the patient show where the pain is?
- Appearance – posture, tension of facial muscles?
- Local signs – swelling, bruising, inflammation, deformity of joints?

Mild pain may be amenable to self-medication with simple analgesics, such as paracetamol. Localised pain from a wound may be relieved once it is dressed; or from an abscess once it is drained. Referral to the doctor will be necessary for patients with more severe pain.

Trauma

A practice nurse who treats a patient following an injury has a duty to ensure that the patient receives the most appropriate advice and treatment. A doctor should be consulted if there is any doubt about the diagnosis or management. Whenever a patient sustains a tetanus-prone wound, the patient's anti-tetanus immunisation must be checked and a booster or primary course given if needed. (See Chapter 11, *Immunisation*).

Abrasions

The superficial skin loss caused by friction can be very painful because the sensory nerve endings in the skin are exposed. Thorough cleaning of the wound with water or saline is needed because residual grit can discolour the skin after healing. It may be possible to remove some particles from the wound by using fine splinter forceps. Irrigation with a solution of hydrogen peroxide may loosen finer dirt particles. A suitable non-adherent dressing or occlusive dressing will be needed to protect the wound and promote epithelialisation. (See Chapter 5 *Dressings*).

Lacerations

The arrest of haemorrhage is discussed above. Most simple lacerations can be sutured in the treatment room. In general all wounds which are gaping, especially on the scalp, fingers and over joint surfaces, will need suturing. Some nurses have been taught to suture, and may be authorised to do so in the surgery, within the limits agreed in a protocol.

The use of adhesive steri-strips has reduced the number of injuries which need suturing. Special skin glue can also be obtained, but the expense precludes its regular use in general practice[9]. Steri-strips (GP41) can be purchased, and reimbursement claimed on an FP10.

Burns and scalds

The immediate first aid treatment for a burn or scald is to put the affected area into cold water. Cold immersion considerably reduces the amount of tissue damage produced by heat[10].

If redness only has occurred and the area is small then probably no treatment will be required. Sunburn is commonly seen in the treatment room as a first or even second degree burn. Soothing creams or calamine lotion will be sufficient if blistering has not occurred. A patient with severe sunburn may require analgesics, dressings, antihistamines and possibly steroids.

When blistering occurs, the blisters should be left intact if possible, but may have to be punctured with a sterile needle and the serum expressed. The skin should be left in place to protect the raw area underneath. A suitable dressing should be applied. Occlusive film dressings are useful for superficial burns and scalds. Flamazine cream helps to prevent infection and aid healing. It can be used with non-adherent dressings and occlusive films; or applied to a burnt hand, which is then enclosed in a polythene bag or large polythene glove. Patients who have extensive or deep burns should be treated in hospital.

Soft tissue injuries

More soft tissue injuries are likely to be seen as patients are encouraged to take more exercise[11]. They need to be given advice about sensible exercise for their age and general condition.

Strains and sprains cause swelling, bruising and pain in the affected tissues. The history will usually make the situation clear. Sometimes a fracture may also be suspected and must be treated accordingly. If swelling occurred immediately after the accident, then the patient should probably be referred to hospital for X-rays. Injuries to tendons and ligaments usually take several hours longer to swell. The initial treatment for a soft tissue injury includes:

- **Rest** – to avoid further damage to the tissues.
- **Ice** – to constrict peripheral blood vessels to reduce bruising and oedema, e.g. a small pack of frozen peas applied for 5–10 minutes

3–4 times a day. (Tell the patient to not eat the peas after they have been refrozen.)

- Compression – to reduce the swelling and provide support, e.g. double tubigrip.
- Elevation – to drain oedema by gravity and relieve pain[12].

Patients may be referred to a physiotherapist for treatment.

Fractures

Patients who have an obvious fracture will usually be transported directly to an accident and emergency department. However minor fractures will be presented in the treatment room, usually associated with other trauma such as bruises, sprains or lacerations. Particular care is needed with hand injuries because lasting deformities could result. It is important to check that the tendon has not been affected in a finger injury. If there is any tenderness in the snuff-box area (the hollow between the base of the thumb and index finger) the injury must be treated as a scaphoid fracture until proved otherwise. Failure to recognise a scaphoid fracture can result in litigation for negligence[13].

Some isolated practices may do much more in the way of dealing with trauma, but it is beyond the scope of this book to go into the details of setting fractures and other major casualty work.

Stings and bites

Human and animal bites can often become infected; so the patient may need antibiotics as well as treatment for the wound. Tetanus immunity should be checked, and in the case of human bites, the patient may also require immunisation against hepatitis B. The possibility of rabies should be considered if an animal bite occurred abroad.

Insect bites

Insect bites are usually easy to diagnose as the lesions are single, or in a cluster, and very irritating. Some bites cause a blister to form in the centre of the lesion and these should be burst with a sterile needle and a dry dressing applied. All other bites are best treated with calamine lotion plus antihistamine tablets if the irritation is severe. The possibility of malaria should be considered if a patient returns from a tropical area with mosquito bites.

Wasp and bee stings

Insect stings usually cause pain in the lesion but require little treatment in the majority of cases. A bee may leave the sting behind and this will need to be removed. Grasp the sting horizontally with forceps, below the poison sac, as close to the skin as possible and lift the sting out. Topical applications such as Wasp-Eze spray can provide reassurance and may ease the discomfort. Hydrocortisone cream 1% will help to reduce the local inflammation, and antihistamine tablets will be needed if the reaction is severe.

If a patient is stung in the mouth, ice should be given to suck to reduce the swelling. Transfer to hospital should be arranged if there is any risk of oedema obstructing the airway.

In rare cases of severe allergy, an anaphylactic reaction can occur. Patients to whom this has happened should carry adrenaline injections everywhere with them throughout the summer months, and know what to do in an emergency.

Ticks

These little insects, found in long grass and woodlands, can attach themselves to the skin. They bury their head in the skin and grow in size as they suck blood. It is important to remove the insect without leaving the head still buried. Plaster remover or spirit applied to the tick should make it withdraw backwards. It can then be removed with forceps, by using sideways movements to release the head from the skin. It is important to avoid leaving the head-part behind.

Ticks can cause Lymes disease and encephalitis; so the patient should be told to see his doctor if any fever occurs within the next fortnight, and to mention the removal of the tick.

Foreign bodies

Eye

The eye may be affected by an infection, foreign body, direct force or penetrating injury. A careful examination is needed, and referral for medical treatment, in all but the most straightforward cases.

The history of getting a piece of dust or similar material in the eye will give an important clue to a foreign body. Usually only one eye is affected and that will feel gritty or painful. The eye will be red and probably watering but in simple cases there will be no discharge.

Examine the eye carefully (see Chapter 5). Irrigation of the eye with saline may remove a foreign body. If it can be seen and is not embedded, then it may be possible to remove it with a moistened swab. A foreign body under the eyelid may be dislodged by drawing the upper lid over the lower lid so that the lower eyelashes sweep inside the lid. The upper lid can be everted by gently holding an orange stick across the base of the eyelid while holding the eyelashes with the other hand and quickly drawing the eyelid outwards and upward over the orange stick (Fig. 7.5).

No attempt should be made to remove a foreign body which is stuck or embedded. In such a situation, if no doctor is available, the patient should be referred to the ophthalmic casualty department for treatment. If a foreign body is suspected but not seen, then the eye should be stained with fluorescein. A few drops instilled in the eye will help to identify a foreign body, corneal abrasion, or dendritic ulcer.

Corneal abrasions occur if the cornea is scratched by a foreign body or a finger-nail. Fluorescein stains abrasions yellow/green where epithelial cells have been removed from the cornea. Abrasions need local antibiotic drops for a few days and the patient might need dark glasses.

Dendritic ulcers are caused by a herpes-like virus which can cause considerable damage to the eye if unrecognised. The symptoms are often identical to a foreign body – pain and a red eye. However, once stained, the ulcer appears as a tiny branching structure – more like the branches of a tree than the single line or mark of a corneal abrasion. Referral is needed if a dendritic ulcer is found.

Nose

Children are remarkably adept at putting an assortment of items up their noses. The problem may become apparent because the child has

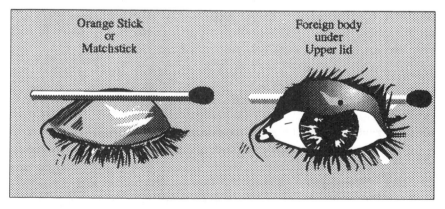

Fig. 7.5 Eversion of the upper eyelid.

obvious difficulty breathing through the nose, or a foul nasal discharge develops.

If an object is small enough to go into the post-nasal cavity it can then fall down into the posterior pharynx and be inhaled into the airway. Thus foreign bodies in the nose should be approached cautiously and the patient be referred to a doctor if the object cannot not be removed easily with nasal forceps.

Ear

A similar assortment of items may be found in the external auditory meatus. It may be possible to remove a foreign body within view with a fine pair of forceps, but if the removal is causing pain or bleeding, then the patient must be referred to the doctor. After removal of the object the drum and meatus should be examined carefully to exclude unexpected damage to them.

Vagina

A woman may be too embarrassed to consult a male doctor, so a female nurse could be asked to retrieve a lost tampon. A vaginal examination should be performed, and it may be possibly to ease the tampon out if it can be felt easily. Often it is necessary to pass a vaginal speculum and use long forceps to retrieve the object from the vaginal vault.

Emergency midwifery

Although there would usually be time to summon help or transfer the patient to hospital, a nurse could be called upon to deliver a baby in exceptional circumstances. For anyone without midwifery experience, the *First Aid Manual* has a good description and illustrations of what to do in an emergency[14]. This book is recommended for reference in all the situations which require first aid.

Suggestions for evaluation and research

- Review your professional profile and emergency equipment:
    - (a)   How well-equipped do you feel to provide first aid or emergency treatment?
    - (b)   What further training or resources do you require?
- Audit the number of occasions you dealt with emergency situations or gave first aid over a chosen period of time:

    (a)   In how many did you discuss the cause of the incident and ways to avoid similar problems in the future?

    (b)   What was the outcome of those incidents dealt with exclusively by the nurses? Was anything overlooked?

● Devise a questionnaire to find out the circumstances under which a patient would choose to go either to an accident department or to the GP surgery.

References

1. Department of Health (1992) *The Health of the Nation: A Strategy for Health in England*. HMSO, London.
2. Skeet, M. (1981) *Emergency Procedures and First Aid for Nurses*. Blackwell Scientific Publications, Oxford.
3. St John's Ambulance, St Andrew's Ambulance Association, British Red Cross (1992) *First Aid Manual* (6th Edn). Dorling Kindersley, London.
4. European Resuscitation Council (1992) *Instructors' Guide*. UK Resuscitation Council.
5. St John's Ambulance, St Andrew's Ambulance Association, British Red Cross (1992) *First Aid Manual* (6th Edn): 73. Dorling Kindersley, London.
6. Ibid: 121.
7. Lowdon, I., Briggs, M. and Cocklin, J. (1989) Head Injury; *Injury*, **20**(4): 193–194.
8. Royal College of Nursing (1992) *Diabetes Clinical Guidelines for Practice Nurses*. Bayer Diagnostics.
9. Gulliver, G. (1991) Sticking together; *Nursing Times, (Journal of Wound Care Nursing)* **87** (5 June): 74–78.
10. Cason, C. (1993) The burning question; *Practice Nursing*, 1–14 June: 13.
11. Holmes, D. (1992) Injury prevention: why warm-ups are cool. Report on sports medicine; *Practice Nurse*, **5**: 233–234.
12. Bird, H. (1991) Sports injuries and their management; *Practice Nurse*, **4**: 355–388.
13. Hooper, G. (1990) Early management of common fractures and dislocations; *Update*, **40**(3): 223–229.
14. St John's Ambulance, St Andrew's Ambulance Association, British Red Cross (1992) *First Aid Manual* (6th Edn): 189–195. Dorling Kindersley, London.

Further reading

Basket, P. (1993) *Resuscitation Handbook* (2nd Edn). Wolfe, London.
Walsh, M. (1990) *Accident and Emergency Nursing – A New Approach* (2nd Edn). Butterworth Heinemann, Oxford.

Useful addresses

Royal Society for the Prevention of Accidents
Cannon House,
Priory Queensway,
Birmingham.
Telephone 021-200 2461.

Chapter 8
Common Medical Conditions

A practice nurse may be consulted about a variety of common conditions. Some will be self-limiting illnesses, like colds and gastric upsets, for which advice can be offered on the management of symptoms. Other problems will obviously require referral to the doctor. The doctor has the ultimate responsibility for medical treatment, so one should always refer if in any doubt.

The hidden agenda

Patients who attend frequently with seemingly minor problems may be looking for a chance to discuss a deeper worry. It is the responsibility of the doctor or nurse to provide the patient with a suitable opportunity to ventilate other problems, especially if the consultation seems inappropriate for the symptoms presented.

Medication

The number of effective drugs available for purchase in a pharmacy changes periodically, and many more have become available since the introduction by the Department of Health of the restricted prescribing list which prohibited many commonly prescribed medications from being prescribed on an FP10. Some drugs can only be prescribed by their generic names[1]. Nurses may be asked for advice about suitable over-the-counter (OTC) medicines, so it is essential to enquire about any allergies, other medication, possible pregnancy or other medical conditions before recommending proprietary products. As cost is a major factor for patients on low income, prescriptions may need to be issued for those who are exempt from prescription charges. Information should be available in the surgery about help with NHS costs[2]. Pharmacists will advise patients about a wide range of problems and treatments. A friendly pharmacist is also a valuable source of information for doctors and nurses.

The practice nurse's responsibility regarding prescriptions

- To ensure that any prescription requested by the nurse is given to the correct patient.
- To be able to answer knowledgeably, or refer to the appropriate person, any enquiries by patients about their medication.
- To ensure that no abuse of drugs occurs in the area of responsibility of the nurse; also that no prescription pads in the nurses' rooms are accessible to patients.
- To be familiar with the repeat prescribing system.
- To have appropriate reference material available.

Reference books

The three main books to have at hand:

(1)   The *British National Formulary* (*BNF*) – a small book packed with information about the commonly used drugs, their indications and contraindications and a guide to their use. It is issued free to all general practitioners via the FHSA.

(2)   The *Monthly Index of Medical Specialties* (*MIMS*) – a comprehensive list of proprietary preparations available on prescription or 'blacklisted'. There is a brief outline of indications and contraindications, plus detailed information on prescribing and cost. It is issued independently and financed by drug advertising. There is no indication of which drug or preparation is more useful than another. *MIMS* is distributed free to all general practitioners monthly and contains information about new products.

(3)   The *OTC Directory – Treatment for Common Ailments* – produced by the Proprietary Association of Great Britain is a valuable reference book on products available without prescription. It is not comprehensive, as companies pay for their products to be included. The format is similar to that of *MIMS* except there that are colour illustrations of all the products in the *OTC Directory*. It is distributed with *MIMS*.

If patients are given advice by nurses on self-management they must be told to consult their GP if the condition worsens or does not resolve in the time expected. Verbal information is forgotten quickly, so important points can be reinforced with printed handouts or leaflets.

It is possible to give only a brief overview of some of the medical conditions with which practice nurses may be involved. So much depends on the circumstances in individual surgeries and the experience of the nurses concerned.

Upper respiratory tract infections

The majority of upper respiratory symptoms due to infection are caused by viruses. Antibiotics may only be required if secondary bacterial infection supervenes. Advice to patients should include:

- An explanation of the nature of viral infections.
- The value of analgesic/antipyretic compounds, such as aspirin or paracetamol, in appropriate dosage. (Aspirin is not recommended for children under 12 years[3].)
- Suggestions about proprietary cough linctuses and decongestants. (Remember to warn patients that antihistamines in some preparations can cause drowsiness. Hypertensive patients should avoid nasal decongestants, which can raise blood pressure.)
- The need for regular drinks to prevent dehydration.
- Advice about the environment:
    (a) bedrest is not necessary unless the patient feels more comfortable there,
    (b) central heating and crowded, smoky atmospheres can make symptoms worse,
    (c) if apyexial the only value in being away from work is to avoid passing the infection on to other people.
- To consult the doctor if:
    (a) a fever persists,
    (b) the sputum becomes discoloured (antibiotics may be required),
    (c) there is pain on inspiration (could indicate pleurisy),
    (d) earache or facial pain occur (could indicate infection of the ears or sinuses).

Smokers may be receptive to offers of help to quit while symptoms make them disinclined to smoke.

Catarrh

The term *catarrh* covers a multitude of disorders related to the sensation of congestion in the nasal airways and sinuses. Some patients suffer all the time (with perennial rhinitis or chronic sinusitis); others may have an acute problem related to hay fever or the common cold. The treatment will depend on the underlying cause. The patient's occupation should always be recorded because there may be an acquired sensitivity to fumes, dust or chemicals at work.

Seasonal rhinitis (hay fever)

The symptoms of hay fever: itchy, watering eyes, sneezing, blocked or running nose, and sometimes wheezing chest, are caused by an allergic reaction to pollen or mould spores. Atopic individuals have an inherited tendency to develop hay fever, asthma and eczema. Changes in farming practices can affect pollen levels[4]. Atmospheric pollution is thought to be a co-factor by causing mucosal damage, which makes sensitisation to allergens easier[5].

Patients known to suffer from seasonal rhinitis are advised to start preventive therapy a fortnight before the hay fever season begins[6].

Treatments available

(Some treatments are not suitable for children.)

- *Antihistamines* – terfenadine (*Triludan*) available OTC, and loratadine (*Clarytin*) are examples of the newer antihistamines which do not cause drowsiness. With products like chlorpheniramine (*Piriton*) and promethazine (*Phenergan*), patients must be warned against driving or working with machinery.
- *Mast cell stabilisers* – sodium cromoglycate as eye drops (*Opticrom*), nasal spray (*Rynacrom*), or inhaler (*Intal*) as preventive treatment.
- *Steroids* – beclomethasone (*Beconase*), budesonide (*Rhinocort*), fluticasone (*Flixotide*), flunisolide (*Syntaris*) nasal sprays.
  Long acting steroid injections may occasionally be prescribed.

Perennial rhinitis

Although the symptoms and treatment are similar to hay fever, people with perennial rhinitis suffer the symptoms all year. Instead of pollen they may be sensitive to allergens like house dust mites or animals. Nasal polyps should be ruled out as a cause of symptoms.

Ear conditions

A practice nurse should learn to visualise the external meatus of the ear and the tympanic membrane, and be familiar with the appearance of a normal drum. Children in particular are susceptible to middle ear infections following a cold and any child who complains of earache should be examined. If a practice nurse examines the ears and the drums are not absolutely normal then the child should be referred to the doctor for advice. Children with ear problems require adequate treatment to prevent hearing loss, which can affect their education[7]. Practice nurses can help to ensure parents understand the importance of compliance with treatments prescribed.

Deafness

'Blocked ears' may be caused externally by excessive wax, debris from otitis externa, or foreign bodies and internally by congestion of the middle ear. Ear syringing should only be performed for the removal of wax in uncomplicated cases (see Chapter 5). In all other circumstances the patient should be referred to a doctor. Decongestants such as pseudephadrine may be recommended for congestion of the middle ear if the patient is otherwise well.

Eye conditions

(See Chapter 5, *Eye treatments*.)
   Patients may present with painful red eyes, and as the range of conditions possible is so great, the nurse must refer to a doctor if in any doubt whatsoever.

Conjunctivitis

This is a common condition with a variety of causes. The signs are:

- A painful or 'gritty' red eye with inflammation across the conjunctiva making the eye look pink. One or both eyes may be affected.
- Discharge that may be purulent or just excessive tears.
- The vision is unaffected.

The important differential diagnosis for conjunctivitis is to exclude a foreign body from the surface of the eye. If a foreign body is suspected, but not seen on examination then the eye should be stained with fluorescein drops to help identify a foreign body, corneal abrasion, or dendritic ulcer (see Chapter 7).
   All other causes of conjunctivitis are usually infective or allergic. Very young babies often get conjunctivitis or a purulent discharge from the

eye when they get an upper respiratory tract infection. This is because the tear duct system is often not fully developed until the baby is about six months old. A few blocked tear ducts eventually require surgery. Advice may be needed on how to clean discharging eyes.

One should always bear in mind the rare case of gonococcal conjunctivitis in the newborn or very young, as this is an extremely serious infection which needs urgent treatment of mother and child.

Other causes of painful eyes

Of the many other causes of painful eyes which require referral, acute glaucoma is probably the most significant. In this condition the intra-occular pressure rises, the cornea is often hazy, vision is poor and the patient is in pain. This is an emergency, as sight is rapidly lost. Chronic glaucoma is more common but does not usually present acutely. The onset is more insidious, possibly with headaches, but treatment is necessary to prevent loss of vision.

Herpes zoster (shingles) may present as pain in the eye or forehead before the typical eruption starts. Once the vesicles begin to develop the diagnosis is obvious and the patient should be referred for treatment urgently.

Headache

Patients with occasional headaches usually treat themselves with OTC analgesics. Most causes of headache are minor, but more serious disease has to be eliminated. Patients with headaches sometimes refer themselves to the practice nurse for a blood pressure check. A medical assessment should be arranged for a patient with recurrent or severe headaches, but once serious disease has been ruled out, the practice nurse can help the patient to deal with the symptoms and to devise avoidance strategies.

Migraine

There are several theories to explain the symptoms of migraine. The cause is still not fully understood[8]. Episodic attacks of severe uni-lateral headache, nausea or vomiting, photophobia or other neurological disturbances lasting for several hours or days are characteristic. Attacks can be preceded by a visual or sensory disturbance (aura) and migraine is now classified as *migraine with aura* and *migraine without aura*[9]. About 70% of sufferers have a family history of migraine. A number of trigger factors – dietary, hormonal, emotional and environmental, are implicated and sometimes an accumulation of triggers will precipitate an attack. No diagnostic test exists, so a clear history of symptoms is needed. A migraine diary can aid diagnosis and help patients to identify possible trigger factors.

Treatment

There is no cure but drugs can sometimes be effective in preventing or relieving symptoms. Changes in lifestyle to avoid trigger factors, relaxation techniques and alternative therapies like acupuncture can be beneficial. Some nurses are involved in migraine clinics with an holistic approach to the problem[10]. The association for Migraine in Primary Care Advisers encourages migraine management in general practice. Self-help groups also exist for sufferers.

Tension headaches

The sensation of a tight band around the head caused by tension in the neck muscles, can be eased by relaxation, stress reduction and massage. Analgesia may also be required.

'Hangover'

Headache following excessive alcohol intake is not uncommon. Practice nurses can give information to sufferers on sensible drinking (see Chapter 9) and advise on the prevention of 'hangover' by maintaining adequate hydration.

Insomnia

Doctors are often requested by patients to prescribe something 'to help me sleep'. Many patients have a high expectation of a perfect night's sleep irrespective of age, other concomitant illness or their own personal needs. A great deal more is known now about sleep and the way various drugs affect it, and doctors are more reluctant to prescribe drugs likely to cause addiction or habituation.

Nurses may be able to help patients who are having difficulty in sleeping. Thorough assessment of the problem may present possible solutions:

- *Daytime sleep*. An elderly patient who has several short naps during the day will not sleep so well at night or need to do so.
- *Pain*. People with severe pain sometimes request sleeping tablets, when adequate analgesia would be more effective.
- *Mental distress*. Counselling may be offered to patients with anxiety or other distress. People with severe depression could require treatment with anti-depressants.
- *Nocturia*. This merits investigation for urinary infection, diabetes, prostatism or the timing of diuretics.

Considering the sleeping environment – a warm milk drink, reading in bed and comfortable bedding all encourage the mind and body to wind down from the day's activities. Relaxation techniques can be taught. Quietness may take more innovation to achieve, especially if a partner snores. Ear plugs may provide relief, and ENT assessment of the snorer may be possible.

Gastro-intestinal disorders

Diarrhoea and vomiting are common symptoms, particularly in children. While most of these episodes are relatively trivial and self-limiting, the risk of dehydration or the masking of more severe pathology, such as intestinal obstruction, has always to be borne in mind.

Causes

The causes of diarrhoea and vomiting are many. Age is an important consideration when trying to decide about likely cause and future management. Some of the major causes in order of frequency are:

Vomiting

- viral, bacterial or toxic causes in all age groups,
- feeding problems in babies,
- pregnancy,
- Meniere's disease or labyrinthitis in middle-aged and elderly, particularly if there have been previous episodes,
- migraine,
- middle ear or upper respiratory infection in childen,
- intestinal obstruction, particularly in babies and the elderly.

Diarrhoea

- following vomiting, almost always infective and often viral,
- on its own at any age, infections, occasionally from contaminated food. Enquire about recent travel,
- other bowel disorders such as ulceratice colitis. The length of history will usually give the clue to these conditions,
- spurious diarrhoea in the elderly, caused by faecal leakage around impacted faeces.

Management

In simple, uncomplicated cases where the patient is over one year of age and the history is only a matter of hours, then frequent small sips of fluid, starvation until bowel symptoms have subsided are all that is required.

Advise the patients to contact the practice again if symptoms persist more than 24 hours or if abdominal pain is persistent or severe.

Children under a year old or any patients whose symptoms do not fit into the infective pattern should be referred to the doctor the same day.

Patients with diarrhoea who work as food handlers should have stool samples sent for culture and be advised to stay away from work until shown to be free of infection.

Dyspepsia

Probably more OTC remedies are bought for indigestion than for most other symptoms. Causes can include poor eating habits, pregnancy, hiatus hernia, smoking and high alcohol consumption. However clinical diagnosis is difficult and patients with persistent symptoms will require medical investigations. The nurse may be the first person consulted, so any patient taking antacids regularly, having a lot of pain, or loss of weight needs referral.

Constipation

Patients can become anxious if their bowels do not work regularly, as witnessed by the many tons of laxatives consumed annually. Normal bowel habits vary, so a diagnosis of constipation has to be related to the norm for each individual. The advice given will depend on the age group of the patient. However the possibility of intestinal obstruction should be considered when a patient has severe constipation. A thorough history must be taken before any advice or treatment is offered.

Babies

Babies often become constipated when their dietary intake is being changed, e.g. change from breast to bottle or milk to solids. Simple reassurance together with an increase in the amount of fluid given (not just milk) may be all that is required.

Young children

Young children may be slow to acquire normal toilet training habits. Health visitors will advise parents about toilet training. It is important not to focus too much attention on bowel function because a child can learn to exert power over parents by refusing to comply.

Children can also be so absorbed in their daily activities that they forget to go to the toilet and so become constipated by suppressing the normal bowel reflexes.

Fear of defecation can result from the experience of passing a painful stool or from an anal fissure.

Management of constipation in children

Advise the parents to increased the roughage in the diet (fruit puree, vegetables, high-fibre cereals and bread), and to introduce extra fluids.

Encourage regular, unhurried toileting after a meal and reward the child with praise.

The doctor may prescribe faecal softeners (e.g. Dioctyl) and/or paediatric glycerine suppositories to relieve severe constipation; and lignocaine anaesthetic gel to be applied around the anus to assist a child to pass a painful motion.

Adults

Constipation in adults or the elderly may be acute or chronic. Acute constipation can be the result of activity restriction by illness or injury, dehydration or drugs such as codeine. Long-term laxative use can cause chronic constipation. The bowel loses its muscle tone and reflexes, so a vicious circle is created whereby the bowel only functions when stimulated by purgatives.

Poor diet and lack of exercise contribute to constipation in all age groups. Changes in bowel habits can be a sign of significant bowel disease, so constipation in a patient who has previously been regular; or alternating constipation and diarrhoea, requires medical investigation.

Management of acute constipation

First, identify the cause if possible and ask for a medical examination if necesssary.

Second, deal with the immediate problem. Advise on the use of simple laxatives or glycerine suppositories in mild cases.

Third, advise on the prevention of a recurrence by the use of softening agents, increased fibre and fluids. If patients have to take drugs known to cause constipation, suitable laxatives will need to be prescribed as well.

Management of chronic constipation

First, encourage gradual re-education of the bowel with changes in diet to increase fibre and fluids.

Second, change the patient's use of stimulant laxatives to faecal softeners and bulking agents.

Encouraging patients to change the habits of a lifetime requires patience. Sudden increases in dietary fibre can cause distressing flatulence, which patients should be warned to expect and be reassured that the problem will settle once the body adjusts.

Worms

Harmless threadworms are the most common parasitic worms which inhabit the gut in the UK, especially in children. Roundworms and tapeworms are less common, but can cause anorexia, weight loss and abdominal distension. Travellers may occasionally return with other helmintic infestations.

Threadworms

Threadworms, true to their name, look like small white threads. They inhabit the bowel and emerge at night to lay their eggs around the anus, causing intense irritation which can disturb sleep or cause bed-wetting.

Treatment should include all the family. Anthelmintic preparations can be bought over the counter or prescribed by the GP. Piperazine can be given to children from one year of age (in a lower dose for children under six). Mebendazole is only suitable for children over two, but in the same dose for all age groups. The nurse has a role in teaching parents how to avoid re-infestation. Information leaflets are available from local Health Promotion Departments.

Threadworms are spread by ingestion of the eggs from hand contact. Scratching the perianal skin will transfer eggs to the hands. Prevention therefore depends on hand hygiene, keeping finger-nails short, and family members using their own face flannels and towels.

Urinary problems

Cystitis

The complaint of cystitis may mean anything from slight burning or frequency of micturition to severe pain, nausea and febrile illness. Cystitis is very common in women, and may or may not be associated with a proven urinary tract infection. Inflammation of the lower urinary tract is often associated with sexual intercourse. Changes in cell structure due to loss of oestrogen can make post-menopausal women prone to cystitis. Organisms which colonise the bowel will cause infection if they gain entry to the bladder. Anatomical differences make this much less common in men; an underlying cause should be sought for any man who has symptoms of cystitis.

Most urinary tract infections will be picked up with diptests for nitrites, leucocytes, blood and protein[11]. A midstream specimen of urine may be sent for microbiology. Antibiotics will be required to treat confirmed urinary tract infections. Women who are prone to recurrent attacks of cystitis can be given information on ways to minimise problems:

- Wipe from front to back after using the toilet, to avoid bringing bowel organisms in contact with the urethra.
- Avoid using scented soaps, bath products, talc and vaginal deodorants, which can irritate the skin.
- Increase fluid intake to about four litres/day.
- Empty the bladder regularly and completely. Wait a few moments then try and empty the last few drops.
- Avoid restrictive clothing and tights, and wear cotton underwear in preference to nylon.
- Use a lubricant if intercourse is affected by vaginal dryness.
- If using a diaphragm, ensure it is the correct size, to avoid pressure against the urethral wall.
- Empty the bladder after sexual intercourse, to flush out any micro-organisms that might have entered the urethra.
- Consult the doctor about hormone replacement for treatment of post-menopausal urinary symptoms.
- If symptoms of cysitis begin, take an alkali – either a proprietory preparation from the chemist or a teaspoon of bicarbonate of soda in

water hourly for three hours; plus 500ml of liquid every 20 minutes for the same length of time.

Cystitis in children

The situation with children is quite different. Undiagnosed infection, often due to an anatomical abnormality, can lead to low-grade pylone-phritis with no symptoms, which can ultimately cause renal failure. Therefore it is vital to examine the urine of children and refer to the doctor if there is the slightest chance of a urinary infection being present. Surgery may be necessary to correct some urinary tract abnormalities.

Inefficient development of the valves at the ureto-bladder junction will allow reflux of urine up the ureters on micturition. If they can be kept free of infection, most children develop the use of these valves by eight to ten years of age. Therefore antibiotic treatment may be required for several years, with MSUs about every three months. A partnership is needed for successful long-term treatment and the prevention of renal damage. Practice nurses can provide support and education and encourage compliance with the medication.

Other causes of cystitis in children include vaginal infection or balanitis, foreign body, and worms. The possibility of sexual abuse also has to be borne in mind.

Vaginal discharge

Many women have varying amounts of vaginal discharge present, either at certain times of the menstrual cycle or all the time. Infection can be caused by a variety of organisms, often sexually transmitted. Offensive discharge may result from a forgotten tampon or other foreign body. It is important to establish exactly what a woman is complaining about when she says she has a vaginal discharge. A high vaginal swab will usually be required to identify the cause of infection.

Candida albicans (thrush)

If the normal balance of commensal organisms is disturbed, an over-growth of yeasts can result. Antibiotics, diabetes, pregnancy and the oral contraceptive are some of the contributary factors. The characteristic white cheesy discharge of candida infection is very irritant. Treatment is usually simple and consists of antifungal vaginal preparations as pessaries or cream. Clotrimazole (*Canesten*) is now available over the counter. Oral treatment, one capsule of fluconazole (*Diflucan*), can be prescribed for more intractable cases. The nurse can explain the condition to patients and advise on ways of preventing a recurrence:

- Avoid using scented soaps, talc etc.
- Wear loose-fitting cotton underwear.
- Wear stockings instead of tights.
- Avoid tight-fitting jeans and trousers.
- Avoid strong detergents.
- Avoid coloured toilet paper.

Bacterial vaginosis

Bacterial infections of the vagina can also cause an irritating discharge. Sometimes patients request a repeat of treatment for thrush, when the problem is in fact bacterial. A high vaginal swab should be sent when necessary. Most offending organisms can be treated with metronidazole (*Flagyl*).

Trichomonas vaginalis

Trichomonas is sexually transmitted by a flagellate organism and produces a frothy yellow discharge. Metronidazole taken orally for a week will provide effective treatment, but patients must be warned to avoid alcohol totally while taking it. Patients may also require persuasion to persevere with the treatment because it can cause such an unpleasant taste in the mouth, and nausea. Metronidazole suppositories may be prescribed instead.

Chlamydia

Another protozoa, Chlamydia is a common cause of resistant vaginal discharge and pelvic inflammatory disease; although many other carriers are asymptomatic. Special swabs are required to identify the organism. Recognition and adequate treatment with antibiotics is essential because of the serious risk to future health and fertility.

General advice

Patients may have more than one sexually transmitted infection and referral to a genito-urinary clinic will sometimes be advisable. Unfortunately, the former stigma associated with these clinics may deter some patients. A practice nurse can help by explaining the skilled diagnosis and treatment available at specialist centres and by giving practical information about clinic times and location. Appropriate advice may also be given on hygiene, 'safe sex', contraception, and cervical screening.

Infectious diseases

Many of the most common childhood illnesses can now be prevented by immunisation. Patients may contact the practice nurse for information about the risk of contracting or spreading a disease, or for diagnosis of a skin rash. If the nurse takes every opportunity to see rashes presenting in the surgery and to be reminded of their cause and salient features, it will be possible to identify the common conditions and give appropriate advice.

Measles

The child is unwell and has usually been so for several days. He or she is catarrhal with a hard non-productive cough and a temperature of about 39°C. The eyes are often red and there is a blotchy, flat rash over the trunk, head and limbs. The rash often starts behind the ears and will slowly develop over the ensuing 24 hours. Koplik's spots look like tiny white grains of salt on the mucous membrane of the mouth and appear before the rash. They are thus a useful diagnostic pointer when measles is suspected.

Treatment is symptomatic unless secondary infection such as middle ear inflammation supervenes.

Rubella (German measles)

The rash of typical rubella is much more diffuse than measles and is often very striking on the face. The diagnosis should not be made if the posterior occipital chain of lymph glands cannot be palpated, as many virus infections produce a transient non-specific rash very similar to rubella. The rubella rash lasts for several days whereas the imitative virus infections seldom last more than 24 hours. No treatment is required and children only need to be kept out of contact with known expectant mothers. Girls who did not receive MMR still need to be immunised against rubella even if they are thought to have had the clinical infection, because a firm diagnosis is often in doubt.

Varicella (chicken pox)

The characteristic lesion of chicken pox is a small blister-like spot with clear serous fluid in the centre. There will be many of these scattered over the trunk and face, showing various stages of development from an early red spot, through the vesicular stage to crusting and the formation of a scab. The diagnosis will usually be obvious, especially as chicken pox tends to occur in minor outbreaks of cases. Apart from being febrile and irritable a child is not at risk. Treatment with calamine lotion helps to cool down the irritating spots. An antihistamine such as promethazine will reduce the itch and sedate the patient in more severe cases. It can help to put the child in a tepid bath or add sodium bicarbonate to the water to reduce irritation.

Chicken pox infection in the first trimester of pregnancy can cause severe congenital abnormalities in about 3% of cases and infection at the time of delivery poses a risk to the infant[12]. This should be remembered if a pregnant woman seeks advice about chicken pox; a referral to the doctor may be necessary.

Human parasites

Scabies

Scabies is caused by the allergic reaction to a small arthropod which lays its eggs in burrows just below the surface of the skin. It can only be transmitted by direct, skin contact with an affected person. It causes intense irritation and the classical burrow lesions can usually be found in the web of the fingers or the wrist. Although these are common sites, it must be assumed that the whole skin except the head will be affected. Crusted scabies often occurs in immunocompromised patients. It is extremely contagious and will affect the head and face as well.

Treatment choice depends on the patient's age and medical condition. All contacts should be treated at the same time to avoid re-infestation. After a hot bath apply a scabicide cream or lotion (permethrin or malathion) from neck to toes, paying particular attention to the skin folds. Treatment should be reapplied to hands after hand washing. After 24 hours the whole body can be bathed. Skin irritation continues for several days after treatment. In heavily affected cases a further treatment will be needed after ten days.

Pediculosis capitis (head lice)

Head lice are common in all age groups but are found more often on children. They can occur in even the most scrupulously careful house-hold and can engender concern out of all proportion to their effect.

Head lice are usually first noticed as nits; the eggs which the female louse glues to individual hairs. Newly laid eggs will be close to the scalp, and those further away and white are hatched eggs which progress outwards as the hair grows. The louse itself is very small and difficult to see. It passes from one head to another by contact. If lice are discovered, the parent should inform the school, playgroup, or others in close contact.

All the family members should be treated at the same time if one of them has head lice. A second application may be needed after ten days to kill any lice which hatched after the first treatment. Local policies exist for rotating treatments in an attempt to prevent resistance to insecticides. For this same reason regular preventive use of pediculosides must be discouraged. Education of the public to understand the problem and adopt simple measures like twice-daily thorough combing is a better way of preventing infestation. Ordinary combing will injure the lice so they are unable to breed. Weekly checks of children's hair with a special head lice comb will allow early detection. Pregnant women must avoid using permethrin.

Pediculosis pubis (crab lice)

Body lice are usually found in the pubic hair and are more easily seen than head lice as they are larger (about the size of a pinhead). Infection occurs mainly with sexual contact. Treatment is by application of an appropriate lotion (malathion, carbaryl,), left on for up to 12 hours and then washed off.

Other skin conditions

As the boundary between the individual and the outside world, the appearance of the skin can affect the way a person is treated by society. Skin diseases are rarely life-threatening but they can devastate self-esteem. There is plenty of scope for nurses who develop specialist skills in this field to help patients improve their quality of life. Immunosuppressed patients may develop extensive skin disorders[13].

Acne vulgaris

Puberty is never the easiest time to live through; but to develop acne, just when self-image becomes all important, must rank among the crueller tricks of Nature. Young patients with acne ofen need a lot of support and counselling. They should be encouraged to lead a normal social life, and to avoid using make-up to cover blemishes, as this will block sebaceous glands even more. It is a myth that a diet high in carbohydrate and fats will aggravate the situation[14], but the value of non-greasy foods and fresh fruit should be emphasised for general health reasons.

Preparations used in treating acne aim at reducing the grease in the skin, and the number of blocked sebaceous ducts (blackheads). Benzoyl peroxide has an antibacterial effect and removes the surface layer of skin to unblock the pores. For this reason all keratolytic products can make the skin dry and sore. A light moisturising cream may help if this occurs and treatment may also need to be stopped for a few days.

In severe acne with persistent pustules and spots on the face and shoulders the doctor may prescribe long-term systemic antibiotics – tetracyclines or erythromycin. Apart from their action against bacteria, they have a special action on the cells in the lower layers of the skin to make them less likely to produce pustules. These antibiotics are effective but need to be taken for several months at least.

Dianette is a combined pill containing cyproterone acetate which reduces sebum production in the skin. Although it is effective as a contraceptive it does not have a product licence for this purpose. Dianette is only suitable for women because it works by lowering testosterone levels.

Psoriasis

Psoriasis is a chronic skin condition with various types and degrees of severity. Arthritis is sometimes an associated condition. In the commonest plaque form, the disease is characterised by well-demarcated, scaly, dry, red patches.

Topical treatments like coal tar and dithranol, although effective, can be messy, smelly and stain clothing. Calcipotiol (*Dovonex*) is a non-staining ointment which may be more acceptable for treatment of plaque psoriasis. Emollients as bath additives and soap substitutes should be used every day to hydrate the skin.

Moderate sunlight is often beneficial, although sunburn can exacerbate the condition. There may be periods of remission but the condition frequently flares up in response to stress or other trigger factors. Techniques for stress management may be helpful. If steroid treatments are prescribed, their use should be monitored, because inappropriate long-term use can cause thinning of the skin. The finger tip unit is a simple way of teaching patients how much cream or ointment to use to cover a given area[15] (Fig. 8.1).

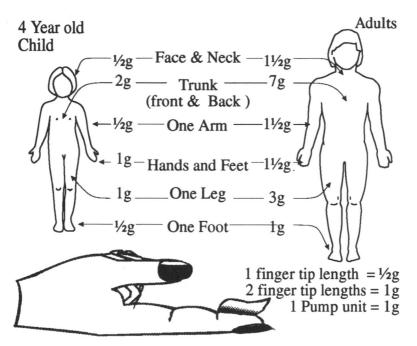

4 Year old Child

Adults

½g — Face & Neck — 1½g

2g — Trunk — 7g
(front & Back)

½g — One Arm — 1½g

1g — Hands and Feet — 1½g

1g — One Leg — 3g

½g — One Foot — 1g

1 finger tip length = ½g
2 finger tip lengths = 1g
1 Pump unit = 1g

Fig. 8.1 Application of steroids – the finger tip unit. (Reproduced with the permission of Glaxo Laboratories Ltd.)

Eczema

The terms *eczema* and *dermatitis* are essentially the same, and mean an inflammatory condition of the skin. The skin eruption may be red and weeping in acute eczema or thickened, dry and scaly in chronic stages. The rash usually causes severe itching and can be exacerbated by infection. There are several ways of classifying eczema:

- *Allergic eczema* – caused by sensitisation to an allergen such as nickel, lanolin, rubber or epoxy resins.
- *Irritant eczema* – occurs in response to substances like detergents, chemicals, or dusts. (If eczema is related to the workplace the patient may be entitled to compensation. Information about occupational skin disease can be obtained from the Employment Medical Advisory service).
- *Atopic eczema* – usually starts in childhood and may accompany asthma and hay fever.
- *Seborrhoeic eczema* – clearly defined red lesions with greasy scale, commonly occurs in the scalp, face and other parts of the skin with

concentrations of sebaceous glands; fungal infection is probably involved. HIV positive patients are particularly susceptible.

- *Varicose eczema* – secondary to venous insufficiency. Can be exacerbated by allergic reactions to topical treatments.
- *Pompholyx eczema* – causes small vesicles on the palms and soles of the feet.

Treatment

Whatever the cause of eczema the treatments are often similar. In acute eczema povidone iodine or potassium permanganate soaks may be prescribed for their anti-infective effect and to dry weeping areas of skin. Systemic antibiotics will be required if the eczema is infected. Steroid creams will probably be needed to control the eczema, but should be avoided until any infection is treated because steroids can suppress the local immune response. Tar-based shampoo may be prescribed for treating seborrhoeic eczema, by reducing sebum production; and anti-fungal preparations – to treat fungal infections.

Long-term care requires diligent skin care and avoidance of exacer-bating factors when possible. Evening primrose oil (*Epogam*) may have effective anti-inflammatory properties and interest in now being shown in Chinese herbal medicine[16]. Patients receiving the latter require regular liver function tests.

The nurse's role lies in helping to educate patients and others about the condition and in providing support and practical advice on man-agement. This will include:

- *Hydration of the skin* – with emollient creams such as aqueous cream and emulsifying ointment, and unperfumed bath oils like *Balneum*, *Emulsiderm* or *Oilatum*. (Patients should be warned of the danger of slipping in a bath containing emollients.)
- *Avoiding soaps, perfumes and other irritants*. Cotton gloves can be worn inside rubber or plastic ones to protect the hands from contact.

Information can be supplied about the relevant voluntary agencies.

Herpes simplex (cold sores)

The common lesion caused by the *herpes simplex* virus is the unsightly cold sore. The virus is acquired, often as a child from the parent, and lives in the cells of the mucocutaneous junction of the lips. When resistance is lower the virus proliferates, producing a tingling sensation followed by painful blisters. The blisters weep and crack and then form scabs which heal in about seven days. Once infected, recurrent attacks can occur in response to trigger factors like stress, sunlight, illness or pregnancy. The virus is contagious and can be spread to other people or to other parts of the body. Genital herpes, eye involvement and herpetic infection of eczema are some of the possible complications. Hence the need for education on ways of preventing spread of the virus by:

- scrupulous hand hygiene,
- not kissing or engaging in oral sex when a cold sore is present,
- not sharing towels or utensils,
- not using saliva to moisten contact lenses.

Acyclovir cream (*Zovirax*), used early in the eruption, may help to minimise the effect. It needs to be applied two hourly as soon as the tingling begins to be of real benefit. Zovirax cream can now be bought over the counter.

Herpes zoster (shingles)

Herpes zoster is the eruption of vesicles seen along the line of a somatic nerve, commonly one on the trunk. The cause is the reactivation of the chicken pox virus which has lain dormant in the dorsal ganglion of the nerve for many years. Therefore a person must have had chicken pox at some time in order to develop shingles. On the other hand, contact with the virus in shingles can result in the development of chicken pox in non-immune individuals.

The lesions of shingles have the specific distribution of the cutaneous nerve. They will be unilateral and stop at the midline. Often pain, which may be intense, is the presenting feature a day or so before the rash develops. The vesicles dry up and fade over the course of 10 to 14 days but the pain may persist as post-herpetic neuralgia.

With lesions following the trigeminal nerve, the eye may be seriously affected.

The treatment essentially consists of encouraging the lesions to dry quickly and avoiding secondary infection of them. The pain should be treated with adequate analgesia (usually something stronger than para-cetamol is required) as the incidence of post-herpetic neuralgia seems to be reduced in those whose pain was adequately controlled in the early stages of the disease. Topical application of acyclovir or idoxuridine may be prescribed. In very severe cases, oral acyclovir may be prescribed at the beginning of the rash.

Bacterial skin infections

Boils, carbuncles

Infected hair follicles can develop into very painful swellings as a result of local inflammation and pus formation. Diabetes should always be ruled out, as recurrent skin infections can be a presenting sign. Sometimes antibiotic treatment will be needed; but in many instances, after hot bathing and magnesium sulphate paste dressings, the lesion will discharge spontaneously, or be ready for incision. Carbuncles usually need incision, and a light calcium alginate wick to encourage drainage.

Impetigo

Impetigo, a staphlococcal infection of the skin can cause unsightly, weeping lesions, with a yellowish crust. The face is commonly affected. Muciprocin ointment (*Bactroban*) will usually clear the infection quickly, but strict personal hygiene – careful hand washing, and separate towels, is needed to prevent it being spread.

Fungal infections

Any part of the body may be affected by fungal infections. Babies can develop distressing fungal rashes in the napkin area. Scrupulous skin-care is essential. Sometimes antifungal creams containing hydro-cortisone are needed to treat the inflammation of the skin. Referral should be made to the GP in such instances.

Tinea pedis (athlete's foot)

Fungal infection readily occurs in the moist skin between the toes, causing itching, maceration and painful cracks.

Left untreated, this can allow entry to other organisms, and result in severe infection of the legs and feet. Treatment with imidazole antifungal preparations (see *BNF*) is usually effective, but Terbinafine (*Lamisil*) is useful for intractable conditions and fungal nail infections. Recurrence is likely if patients do not follow these basic foot care measures:

● Wash the feet at least once a day and dry carefully between the toes. Use antifungal treatment if athlete's foot is present.
● Wear clean socks or stockings every day.
● Wear footwear which allows air to the feet.
● Change footwear regularly.

- See your doctor if the condition does not respond to treatment or the toe-nails become affected.

Warts

Warts are caused by different types of human papilloma virus. Warts on the hands and feet usually disappear spontaneously as the body develops immunity to the virus. Unfortunately this can take many months and patients with unsightly warts on the hands, or pressure symptoms from verrucae, are unlikely to want to wait. Plantar warts (verrucae) are very common in children but schools will sometimes try to exclude a child from swimming or games. Although unlikely to limit the spread, verruca socks can be worn to satisfy the school rules.

If treatment is requested, topical preparations of salicylic acid or glutaraldehyde can be recommended or prescribed. The manufacturer's instructions must be followed. The paint is applied daily, taking care to avoid the surrounding skin. A pumice stone or emery board must be used between applications to remove dead skin. Patients need to persevere with the treatment for up to six weeks. If there is no response minor surgery may be considered.

Genital warts

Genital warts are transmitted sexually and can spread rapidly. They are often associated with other sexually transmitted diseases, so it is recommended that patients are referred to the genito-urinary medical clinic for screening and contact tracing. Women infected with genital wart virus are at particular risk of developing cervical cell changes, so need regular screening.

Warts can be treated in the surgery with podophyllin compound paint by doctors or nurses trained in its use. (Podophyllin must not be used on pregnant women because it is cytotoxic.)

Suggestions for evaluation and research

- Review your job description, professional profile, *Standards of Professional Conduct*, and protocols for work:
    - (a) Do you feel competent to deal with the common medical conditions you encounter in your practice?
    - (b) How does your role as a nurse differ from that of a doctor in those instances?
- Conduct a literature search on the role of practice nurses in the care

of patients with either migraine, or skin diseases. How might this information affect your own practice?

- Audit the times you gave advice to patients about minor medical conditions:
  - (a) How much medical time was saved?
  - (b) How many patients were referred to the GP?
  - (c) How many patients requested a consultation with a nurse instead of a doctor?
- Devise a study to find out what patients understand about the self-management of self-limiting conditions. Use this information with other members of the primary health care team to prepare an education package for the public.

References

1. (a) NHS England and Wales (1988) Statutory Instrument No. 1106. *The National Health Service (General Medical and Pharmaceutical Services) Amendment Regulations 1988.* (b) *NHS (General Medical and Pharmaceutical Services) Amendment Regulations 1990.*
2. Department of Health (from April 1993) *NHS Prescriptions – How to get them Free*; DOH leaflet P11.
3. Mann, R.D. (1986) Reye's Syndrome and aspirin; *Journal of the Royal College of General Practitioners,* **36**, September: 418–421.
4. Bryan, J. and Illman, J. (1993) Why oilseed rape is not to be sneezed at; *The Guardian,* 25 May.
5. Lewith, G. (1993) Pollen perils work in the asphalt jungle; *Doctor,* 6 May: 52–54.
6. Emberlin, G. (1992) Avoiding the perils of pollen; *Practice Nurse,* **5:** 213–216.
7. Mead, M. (1991) Treating chest, throat and ear infections; *Practice Nurse,* **4:** 362–364.
8. Hibbert, A. (1994) Migraine; *Practice Nursing,* 18 January–7 February: 13–14.
9. Martynoga, A. (1993) Migraine: diagnosis and treatment; *Practice Nursing,* 6–19 April: 25–26.
10. Spittal, H. (1993) Migraine management in general practice; *Practice Nursing,* 20 April–3 May: 23.
11. Pritchard, V. and Levernier, J. (1991) Multistix versus laboratory urinalysis in the detection of urinary tract infection; *Journal of Gerontological Nursing,* **17**(8): 39–42.
12. Gilbert, G.L. (1993) Chicken pox during pregnancy; *British Medical Journal,* **306:** 1079–1080.
13. Anastasi, J.K. and Rivera, J. (1992) Identifying the skin manifestations of HIV; *Nursing,* **22**(11): 58–61.

14. Mead, M. (1991) Preparations for skin disorders; *Practice Nurse*, **3:** 637.
15. Long, C.C. and Finlay, A.Y. (1991) The finger tip unit – a new practical measure; *Clinical and Experimental Dermatology*, **16:** 444–447.
16. Sadler, C. (1992) Time for tea? *Nursing Times*, **88**, 26 May: 34–36.

Further reading

Sachs, O. (1991) *Migraine* (2nd revised Edn.) Faber & Faber, London.
Lander, M. (Ed.) *The Medical Management of Insomnia in General Practice.* Royal Society of Medicine, London.
Alderman, C. (1989) Not just skin deep; *Nursing Standard*, **3**, 10 June: 22–23.

Useful addresses

Insomnia Self-Help Group
10 Barley Mow Passage, Chiswick, London W4 4PH.

The British Migraine Association
178a High Road, Byfleet, Surrey KT14 7ED.

The Migraine Trust
45 Great Ormond Street, London WC1N 5HD.

The National Eczema Society
4 Tavistock Place, London WC1 9RA.

The Psoriasis Association
7 Milton Street, Northampton NN2 7JG.

Chapter 9
Health Promotion

The 1990 Contract made GPs responsible for screening and health promotion services for patients of all ages. New arrangements introduced in July 1993, link health promotion to the strategy outlined in the white paper *The Health of the Nation* in which targets are specified for reducing illness and death in five key areas:

(1) *Coronary heart disease and stroke.* To reduce death from CHD and stroke in people under 65 by at least 40% by the year 2000.
(2) *Cancer.* To reduce death from breast cancer in women age 50–64 by at least 25% by the year 2000,
    (a) to reduce the incidence of invasive cervical cancer by at least 20% by the year 2000,
    (b) to halt the annual increase in the incidence of skin cancer by 2005,
    (c) to reduce the death rate for lung cancer by at least 30% in men under 75 and 15% in women under 75 by the year 2010.
(3) *Mental illness.* To reduce the overall suicide rate by 15%, and the rate for severely mentally ill people by at least 30%, by the year 2000.
(4) *HIV/AIDS and sexual health.* To reduce the incidence of gonorrhoea among men and women aged 15–64 by at least 20% by 1995,
    (a) to reduce the rate of conception in girls under 16 by at least 50% by the year 2000,
    (b) to reduce the number of injecting drug misusers who share injecting equipment by at least 50% by 1997, and a further 50% reduction by the year 2000.
(5) *Accidents.* To reduce death from accidents in children under 15 by at least 33% by 2005,
    (a) in people aged 15–24 by at least 25% by 2005,
    (b) in people aged 65 and over by at least 33% by the year 2005[1].

(Scotland, Wales and N. Ireland have similar strategies for health[2].)

Asthma and diabetes care in general practice now attract annual payments, but reimbursement for other clinics has been discontinued. Fees for individual health promotion clinics were replaced by payments in three bands for achieving specific targets[3]. Data has to be collected and help offered to patients for:

- *Band 1* – smoking cessation,
- *Band 2* – reducing morbidity and mortality from hypertension, coronary heart disease and stroke (this includes Band 1 activities),
- *Band 3* – preventing coronary heart disease and stroke. (Includes Bands 1 and 2 activities, as well as primary prevention.)

Terminology

The term *health promotion* is used rather freely nowadays, but its exact meaning warrants some reflection. *Health* is a complex issue; influenced as much by environmental, political, social and genetic factors, as by personal behaviour or lifestyle. *Health promotion* is a broad term covering all those activities which contribute to the social, physical and mental well-being of individuals and societies. In general practice it mainly involves preventive care and health education; although health workers may also campaign for action on the wider issues.

Preventive care aims either to prevent ill-health from occurring, or to keep its effects to a minimum. Three different types of prevention are recognised:

(1) *Primary prevention* covers activities which prevent disease altogether, e.g. immunisation against infectious diseases, encouraging healthy eating and exercise.
(2) *Secondary prevention* aims to detect problems before symptoms develop in order to take remedial action, e.g. child development checks, cervical screening.
(3) *Tertiary prevention* includes the management of existing disease or disability in order to minimise any complications and maximise the patient's quality of life, e.g. reducing high blood pressure to prevent a stroke, maintaining glycaemic control in diabetes.

Screening entails looking for previously unrecognised disease in particular groups of people. Screening tests have to meet various criteria in order to be of value:

- The condition must be treatable.

- It must develop slowly.
- The test must be simple and reliable.
- It must be cost effective in terms of money and manpower[4].

No screening should be undertaken without informed consent. Patients can be subjected to unnecessary investigations and distress if screening tests produce false positive results. Conversely, false negative results may lead patients to ignore subsequent symptoms because of a mistaken sense of security.

Health education seeks to provide learning opportunities about health – either by working with individuals, or generally, through the mass media and advertising. At the personal level health education involves sharing knowledge about health, identifying any risks to health, and helping people to develop the ability to make healthy choices.

Health promotion and the PHC team

Doctors and nurses who undertake health promotion must have discussed the ethical implications and have a clear philosophy of health. Many health behaviours are highly complex; yet there is a danger of attributing blame to people whose actions are perceived as contributing to their own diseases. There must be recognisable benefits based on sound research to justify influencing the health behaviour of others. Some studies have cast doubt on the value of widespread health promotion activities in general practice[5,6]. Hence the need for medical and nursing audit. Doctors and nurses who 'practice what they preach' and act as role models can have greater credibility when they advise their patients about healthy living[7].

Practice nurses have demonstrated their enthusiasm for health promotion, but it cannot be overstressed that individual nurses must be adequately educated for this work. Local Health Promotion units run a variety of training courses and provide support materials. Training in counselling is always valuable and the Health Education Diploma provides a comprehensive grounding. Modules on health promotion can be undertaken at many colleges.

Resources

Better Living – Better Life – a resource book, funded by the NHS Management Executive, covers the lifestyle changes needed for preventing coronary heart disease and stroke[8]. A copy was sent to every practice. It should be a standard reference book for all practice nurses who undertake health promotion. Additional material is needed to cater for the needs of other ethnic groups. The NHS Management Executive is establishing an Ethnic Health Unit to help with the development of services for black and minority ethnic groups[9].

Healthlines – a monthly publication by the Health Education Authority contains topical health-related articles and a digest under subject headings of research and journal articles related to health promotion.

Communication

Communication involves both the transmission and the reception of information or ideas. Non-verbal communication relays messages either consciously or unconsciously, through facial expression, gesture, general appearance and posture. All the senses pick up cues and confusion arises when the non-verbal message conflicts with the spoken one.

Nurses who work in multi-ethnic areas need to be as familiar as possible with the customs of their patients. Problems of communication can occur when a common language or culture is not shared. Interpreters can assist, but the subtle nuances of language will sometimes be lost[10].

A nurse should try to ensure that the information given is meaningful. Written material will be of little use if the patient is illiterate, or cannot see well enough to read. Jargon can be a useful shorthand for those in the know, but is also a way of excluding outsiders. It follows that to use jargon to patients can exclude them too.

It is better to assume nothing and always check what the patient knows and has understood. Many of the techniques of counselling can be used in health promotion:

- *Suitable ambiance.* A quiet, peaceful environment, free from telephone calls and visual distractions will help concentration on the issues.
- *Asking questions.* Closed questions, such as 'do you drink any alcohol?' will elicit short 'yes/no' type answers. Open questions (often beginning with 'what, why, when, where or how') allow a subject to be explored. For example – 'how many days each week do you drink alcohol?' 'What effect do you think this has on your health?'
- *Checking on understanding.* No matter how obvious the message may seem to the nurse, it may be totally obscure to the patient. So it pays to take stock regularly. The nurse can ask the patient to recap in

his/her own words what has been discussed. Alternatively, the nurse may paraphrase what she/he believes the patient has said, to make sure that nothing has been misunderstood.

- *Listening.* It requires a particular skill to be able to sit and give undivided attention to another person; to maintain a calm but attentive posture, to allow eye contact without staring, to give nods of encouragement when needed, but above all – to tolerate pauses without wanting to fill them.

Motivation

Knowledge about health risks alone will not cause people to alter their behaviour[11]. They must feel motivated to change. This means that the rewards of change must outweigh the short-term benefits of the behaviour. Sometimes patients are ambivalent; they want to change but are reluctant to give up the pleasures of their risky behaviour. *Motivational interviewing* is a technique developed by an American psychologist to assist ambivalent people to decide to deal with addictive behaviour[12]. The key points involve:

- *Empathy.* Acceptance of the patient as a person. Trying to enter into the feelings of that person.
- *Developing discrepancy.* Helping the patient to decide to change, and to present his/her own arguments for changing.
- *Avoiding confrontation.* Arguments are counterproductive.
- *Support for self-efficacy.* The patient is responsible for choosing and carrying out personal change.

Health promotion in general practice

Opportunistic health promotion can take place during any consultation or procedure; examples are given in other chapters. The remainder of this chapter deals with planned health promotion activities.

New patient health checks

The 1990 Contract requires all new patients over five years old to be offered a health check, including the measurement of height, weight and blood pressure, and urinalysis for protein and glucose. Such interviews serve several purposes:

- Patients are welcomed to the surgery and given information about the best ways to use the services.

- Essential points about a patient's health are ascertained before the NHS records are transferred. Entries can be made to the disease registers.
- Doctors and nurses can gather details of the patient's social, medical and family history, identify health risks, and offer appropriate help.
- They attract a fee.

Questionnaires can save time, but a face-to-face interview is also needed to clarify the information and to ensure that the patient consents to personal details being recorded. Sensitivity is required, bearing in mind that the patient is in unfamiliar surroundings and may be feeling unwell. The questions need to be appropriate to the circumstances of individual patients. If necessary, a patient can be invited to make another appointment.

Close attention should be paid to the way questions are asked and worded, as it is very easy to give offence. There must be a justifiable reason for asking for information – not just curiosity. Some of the information to be gathered can include the following.

Social background

- *Title.* How would the patient like to be addressed. (This can elicit whether to address a woman as Mrs, Miss, or Ms; or if the patient has some other professional or honourary title.)
- *Household.* Does the patient have someone else at home? This might be a spouse or a lover, another relative, or a lodger. If a patient lives alone it is worth noting the contact address for a relative, in case of a sudden severe illness.
- *Children.* The number and ages of any children may be relevant to the parent's physical or mental health. A check can also be made on the children's immunisation status.
- *Employment.* Are there any occupational hazards to consider? More ill-health and depression could be expected, if unemployed[13]. If a woman has declared herself to be a 'housewife', it is insensitive to ask 'do you work?'; better to enquire about any work outside the home.
- *Smoking.* Never smoked? If an ex-smoker or current smoker – how many a day. How long? – if stopped smoking.
- *Alcohol.* How many units drunk, and over how many days each week?

Past medical history

- *Illnesses.* Any illnesses other than the usual childhood infections.

Cite asthma and diabetes as examples. (Patients do not always think to mention them.)

- *Operations.* List in chronological order.
- *Allergies.* Some patients confuse allergy with side-effects, such as nausea. Any true allergies must be documented prominently.
- *Immunisations.* Patients who have not completed a routine course against tetanus or polio can be offered immunisations.

Current health

- *Any problems?* Ask particularly about indigestion, pain, any abnormal bleeding, or any problems with bladder or bowel function. Consider the possibility of anaemia or thyroid dysfunction.
- *Medication.* What, if any, prescribed or OTC medicines are taken regularly?

(Women only)

- *Parity.* The obstetric history may be relevant to the current health of the patient.
- *Periods.* Questions depending on the age of the patient, regularity, any problems, age at menopause, HRT?
- *Rubella status.* All women who could become pregnant should be immune to rubella. A blood test can be offered, or the patient told of the screening service for the future.
- *Contraception.* Questions as appropriate. Check the method and need for further advice. If the 'pill', how long has the patient been taking it? If an IUD or diaphragm – how long since the last check? If injectable – date of last injection?
- *Cervical smear.* Date and result of the last smear? Any history of abnormal smears/treatment? (Offer a smear appointment if it is due.)
- *Breasts.* Has the patient been taught 'breast awareness'. Has she ever had mammography and if so, what was the result? (Offer advice if appropriate.)

(Men only)

- *Testes.* Has the patient been taught testicular self-examination? Leaflets can be obtained from health promotion departments. The pressure group Save Our Sons campaigns for men to be taught how to detect possible testicular cancers[14].
- *Prostate.* Ask about nocturia or any difficulties passing urine.

Specific questions may detect problems, which men attribute to ageing[15].

- *Other problems.* Men can sometimes be diffident about expressing their feelings or concerns. They may be more willing to seek help when it is needed if a rapport is established during a new-patient interview. Early diagnosis is the key to the successful treatment of many conditions, but men in Britain often postpone seeking help for many months.

Family history

- *Parents and siblings.* Ask particularly about diabetes, CHD, hypertension, stroke, asthma, cancer, glaucoma, thyroid problems, tuberculosis; plus diagnosis and age at death (if no longer alive).

Tests

- *Height and weight.* Calculate the body mass index (weight in Kg divided by height in square metres) from a BMI chart. Check if the BMI is within the normal range (20–25 for men and 18.5–23.6 for women).
- *Blood pressure.* Follow the practice protocol.
- *Urine (glucose).* Screening for diabetes.
- *Urine (protein).* Screening for renal disease or infection. Test for blood, nitrites and leucocytes, or send an MSU if a urinary tract infection is suspected.
- *Peak expiratory flow rate.* If a history of asthma or smoking.

Well-person checks

Although the requirement to offer three-yearly adult screening has been dropped, many patients still request a health check. Landmark birthdays – 40, 50, 60 years, often trigger a sudden interest in health. If a patient asks a nurse for a 'check-up', it is important to identify any particular health concerns and refer to the doctor if necessary. Well-person checks in general practice cover similar ground to that listed above in *New Patient Health Checks*, but the emphasis may vary, depending on the age and sex of the patient. Lifestyle factors – smoking, alcohol consumption, diet and exercise, together with the blood pressure, BMI and any family history, can be used to assess the risks for heart disease, and appropriate help offered. Special CHD risk calculators can be used, with caution[16].

No fee can be claimed for well-person checks, but cervical smears will count towards the target payments, and information on patients aged 16–74 can be collated for the health promotion banding.

Assessment of elderly people

All patients over 75 years have to be offered an annual health check and home visit; which GPs can delegate to other members of the primary health care team[17]. The skills of assessment are included in the education of district nurses and health visitors; practice nurses who undertake home visits, are required by the UKCC to have had comparable training[18]. The Royal College of Nursing has produced booklets dealing with the knowledge and skills needed for assessing the elderly[19,20].

The extent of assessments will be decided within the practice and written into the protocol, but the following points are usually considered.

Social assessment

- *Housing.* Facilities (toilet, bathing, cooking, heating).
    - (a)   Safety. (Any loose rugs/ floorboards, trailing flexes, fire-guards?)
    - (b)   Access. (Stairs, lift, ground-floor?)
- *Carers.* Does the patient live alone? Next of kin? Support from family, friends, warden or social services. Age of carers. Do the carers need more support? Is there evidence of tension in the household; or of abuse of the elderly person?
- *Finance.* Is the patient able to keep warm, buy nutritious food, spend money on luxury items if desired? Are benefits being claimed, if entitled?
- *Lifestyle.* Smoking, alcohol, social contacts, clubs, hobbies?

Physical assessment

- *Ability for self-care* – cooking, bathing, shopping. Condition of skin, hair and nails. Ability to take any medication correctly.
- *Mobility* – indoors and outdoors, stairs. Use of mobility aids, suitability of footwear.
- *Vision* – date of last eye check? Use and condition of spectacles. Ability to read.
- *Hearing* – any difficulty hearing? If patient has a hearing aid – ability to use and maintain it.
- *Dentition* – state of teeth/dentures. Access to a dentist if needed?

- *General health* – sleep, appetite, energy, any pain? Any signs of anaemia or myxoedema?
- *Continence* – any problems with bladder or bowel function? Continence aids/services used or needed.
- *Tests* – blood pressure and urinalysis to detect unrecognised hypertension, UTI or diabetes.
- *Medication* – if any medicines are taken. Does the patient know what they are for and when to take them? Who prescribed them? Are they still in date? Are any duplicated with trade and generic names?

Mental assessment

- *Level of consciousness.* Is the patient alert or drowsy? Ability to concentrate.
- *Mood.* Does the patient appear 'normal', depressed, anxious or elated?
- *Thought and speech.* Does the patient's speech make sense? Is there evidence of hallucinations or delusions?
- *Orientation and memory.* Does the patient know the date; where he/she lives; his/her age? Can the patient remember what was said five minutes ago?
- *Behaviour.* Does it appear appropriate to the circumstances?

A mental assessment can be more difficult than the physical assessment. Patients with dementia can be very plausible, and unless the nurse knows the family well the problem may not always be apparent. A patient can give graphic details of his/her daily activities which relate to years gone by and bear no relationship to the present situation.

Caution

False expectations can be be aroused if situations are encountered for which there are no local services available. Loneliness and problems with bathing and footcare are probably the most common problems, but many social service and chiropody departments are overstretched. Nurses must beware of promising help which cannot be delivered[21].

Dietary advice

Dieticians are responsible for providing specialised dietary advice, but practice nurses are able to give guidance on healthy eating and lifestyles and to monitor patients on diets. Collaboration allows the expertise of dieticians and nurses to be used effectively.

Healthy eating

Food is needed to provide the protein, vitamins and minerals required for healthy tissues, and to supply the energy for daily activity and a normal body weight. Malabsorption, disease and anorexia can cause malnutrition but the majority of the population are more likely to suffer from dietary excess[22]. Most people would benefit from an increase in the consumption of complex carbohydrates and dietary fibre and a reduction in fat, salt and sugar. Fruit and vegetables, wholemeal bread, pasta, rice and cereals should provide the greatest proportion of the diet, with smaller quantities of protein and very little fat[23].

Weight loss

The cause of obesity is simple – more calories are eaten than the body uses up, so the excess is stored as fat. The complexity lies in the reasons for the mismatch. Very few people enjoy being overweight, but strong psychological factors and ingrained behaviour affect their eating habits. Drastic dieting can lead to a rebound weight gain as soon as the will-power fails; therefore the objective must be to help patients to substitute more healthy foods without creating an obsession with the next meal. The following steps can be taken:

- *Obtain a full medical, social and family history* to identify any factors which could affect the patient's weight.
- *Measure the current weight and height* to calculate the body mass index and identify how much weight, if any, needs to be shed.
- *Assess the patient's motivation* to find out if the patient wants to lose weight. Check if he/she perceives the increased health risks of obesity (CHD, diabetes and osteoarthritis). Encourage the ambivalent patient to identify the personal benefits, and positive reasons for change.
- *Set realistic goals.* Small steps which can be reached in a reasonable time will provide the encouragement to persevere because success reinforces motivation[24].
- *Identify the usual eating habits.* Ask the patient to keep an accurate food diary for at least a week. The diary should include the quantities as well as the types of food and drink, and the circumstances when they were consumed. Alcohol consumption should also be recorded. Patients from different cultural backgrounds may eat foods which

are unfamiliar to the nurse. A dietician can be consulted about their nutritional values. More often, the patients may need to be persuaded to avoid the high-fat hamburgers and refined sugars so popular in western diets.

- *Negotiate changes to the diet.* Healthy eating will need to be life-long. Drastic changes to eating habits will not last if the patient does not like the substituted food.

A nurse should be able to offer suggestions in accordance with the patient's income and religious beliefs. Sometimes compromises may be needed to get patients to accept change. For example:

- *Milk.* If skimmed milk is unacceptable, try semi-skimmed. Skimmed milk can be used in sauces and for cooking, where it won't be tasted. Low-fat yoghourt will provide calcium and vitamins if enough milk is not able to be drunk each day.
- *Salads.* Recurrent dieters who hate salads do not have to eat them at all. Alternatively, salad can be used in sandwiches, with hot food, or after the main course as the French eat it. A teaspoonful of low fat salad dressing can make all the difference to the flavour of a salad.
- *Vegetables.* Several different vegetables, even if cooked in the same pot, will be more interesting than a plate loaded with one type. Jacket potatoes make a filling meal with cottage cheese, tuna, baked beans, or yoghourt with onions and herbs (instead of butter).
- *Fruit.* Tinned fruits in fruit juice can be found in most supermarkets. Dried fruits make a delicious snack.
- *Meat.* Smaller quantities of lean meat, skinless chicken or low fat sausages can be grilled, boiled or baked, instead of fried. Poultry is recommended instead because it contains less fat but the skin must be removed before cooking it.
- *Fibre.* If wholemeal bread is not liked, try high-fibre white bread as a start. A few ready-to-eat dried apricots freshly chopped into breakfast cereals will add sweetness and a soft chewy texture. Try mixing different breakfast cereals together for variety of texture and flavour.

After suggesting the above changes for the patient's diet, the practice nurse can then:

- *Monitor progress.* The rapid weight loss of the first weeks will slow down. Particular encouragement is needed when a plateau is reached. Increased physical activity can be advised and keeping a food diary may help to remotivate the patient. New goals can be set as weight is lost.

● *Maintain the target weight.* Once the goal has been reached, adjustments to the diet will be needed to stay at the target weight. Euphoria at having reached the goal can lead the patient to resume the old habits of eating. Throughout the period of weight loss, the benefits of permanent change must be stressed.

Advice about diets should be accompanied by recommendations for appropriate exercise.

Lipid-lowering diets

The public interest in cholesterol has been fostered by the media, but raised cholesterol is only one of a number of contributary factors to coronary heart disease. Moreover, the official view on the importance of cholesterol changes frequently. The selection of patients for testing will depend on the practice policy, but talking to a patient who requests a cholesterol test gives an opportunity for discussing other risk factors – smoking, raised BMI, high alcohol intake, lack of exercise. Help can be given to consider appropriate lifestyle changes. Healthy eating and a strict control of dietary fat is beneficial for everyone, although a minority of patients who have familial hyperlipidaemia, or other medical causes of raised serum cholesterol, may need therapy with lipid-lowering drugs.

Less than 30% of the total daily energy requirement should come from fat, of which not more than 10% should be saturated fat[25]. This will mean little to the average person so it would be better to suggest suitable daily amounts of low-fat spread, salad dressing or oil, and to suggest ways of cooking without fat.

Obvious fats are easier to cope with than the hidden fats in cakes, biscuits and processed foods. The whole subject is a minefield and patients will need to read food labels carefully if they are not to be misled by unrealistic claims on the packet. Low-fat spreads and yoghourts vary considerably in their fat contents. Patients who do not also need to lose weight will have to increase their starchy foods as they reduce their fats in order to maintain their calorie intake.

Better Living – Better Life has a comprehensive chapter on healthy eating and drinking.

Exercise

Some doctors now prescribe 'exercise' in a similar way to prescribing drugs. They have made arrangements with local leisure centres for patients to receive structured exercise[26]. Physical activity has many benefits for health – not least is the prevention of coronary heart disease, and possibly, diabetes[27]. The level of activity must be appropriate for each individual patient. Patients who are obese or have known medical conditions require specialist advice about suitable exercise. The physiotherapist may be willing to advise.

Sensible drinking

Alcohol consumption is an important part of any health assessment. People of all ages have ready access to drink and millions of days are lost each year through drink-related absenteeism. Measurements in units of alcohol makes assessment easier. One unit, equivalent to 8g of pure alcohol, is found in:

$^1/_2$ pint ordinary strength beer
1 single pub measure of spirits
1 small glass of wine.

Sensible drinking is generally considered to be below 21 units a week for men and 14 units for women, spread evenly over the week. Patients who regularly drink more than these amounts need to be made aware of the risks to their health and be offered appropriate help. Alcohol in pregnancy or while breast-feeding can affect the baby, so in such cases women must be advised not to have more than a very occasional drink[28]. Patients with real alcohol dependence, who are willing to seek help, may require medical supervision, or a special support service such as Alcoholics Anonymous. Practice nurses can help patients who want to drink less to agree on a sensible limit and to devise strategies for sticking to it. A drink diary can help the patient to stay within the target limit and to recognise the times and situations when the pressure to drink is greatest. Ways of cutting down which can be suggested include:

- Keep busy to avoid thinking about drink.
- Postpone the first drink until the evening, as late as possible.
- Drink halves instead of pints.
- Try low alcohol drinks instead.
- Dilute spirits with mixers.
- Take small sips and make a drink last.
- Don't get involved in buying rounds.
- Use a measure at home to make sure a drink is only a single, then put the bottle out of sight.

The relationship between drinking and social activities can vary. The importance of not drinking and driving can make the refusal of a drink more socially acceptable, but in other situations peer pressure can be very strong. Sadly, a lot of advertisements seem to be aimed at young people. The money spent on persuading them to drink far outweighs the resources available for health education.

Smoking cessation

There is increasing pressure on smokers to stop. *The Health of the Nation* contains targets for reducing the number of people who smoke as a part of the drive to reduce CHD and strokes. Health professionals are required to identify the patients who smoke, explain the dangers to health and offer them help to stop smoking.

The dangers to health

- heart disease and hypertension
- peripheral vascular disease
- chronic bronchitis and emphysema
- cancer of the lung, throat, mouth and tongue
- cancer of the stomach, pancreas, cervix
- pregnant women are more likely to have smaller, unhealthy babies
- children growing up in an environment where parents smoke are more likely to have respiratory problems
- children follow the example of their parents and peers.

Often patients have symptoms of some of these conditions before they will accept help, but they must be assured that it is never too late to give up smoking and that it can be a very important way of improving health. Younger patients may be more convinced by the social arguments.

Social aspects of smoking

- constant smell of smoke on clothes, body, breath and hair
- cost
- antisocial habit.

It is important to understand the social and psychological pressures which cause people to take up smoking. An information pack is available about working class mothers who smoke[29].

Strategies for quitting

A carbon monoxide monitor can be a useful tool for convincing patients of the effects of smoking. A patient who wants to quit can be helped to devise a plan:

- Work out all the reasons for stopping.
- Decide a date to stop, avoiding a day likely to be stressful.
- Tell people in close contact of the decision, and try to persuade someone else to stop smoking at the same time.
- Decide how to change the routine to avoid the usual triggers for smoking.
- The evening before the 'big' day smoke the last cigarette and then throw away the remaining cigarettes.

Hints for the new non-smoker

- Avoid temptation – put ashtrays, matches and lighters out of sight.
- Keep away from smokers.
- Change habits, avoid breaks when a cigarette is usually smoked. Keep busy.
- Put aside the money saved each day.
- Keep a supply of chewing gum, apple or carrot to nibble if necessary.
- Take more exercise to avoid gaining weight[30].

Nicotine replacement may be useful for nicotine-dependent smokers during the early stages of withdrawal. Nicotine patches, available on private prescription, deliver a measured amount of nicotine transdermally over a 24 hour period. They are not suitable for patients with myocardial ischaemia or for pregnant or breast-feeding women. The manufacturer's instructions should be followed for using the patches and patients should be reminded to remove the old one before applying the next. Nicotine chewing gum (Nicorette) may also be used but the patient needs to understand the technique for 'parking' it in the mouth between chews, instead of constant chewing. Nicorette gum (2mg) can be bought over the counter.

Support for patients

Practice nurses with group leadership skills can run successful support groups for patients who want to lose weight or stop smoking. Alternatively, information may be provided about other locally run groups and support networks. Patients who are changing their behaviour (smoking, drinking or eating) may benefit from supportive therapies. Hypnotherapy or acupuncture can help to reinforce motivation. Stress relieving techniques may be used to reduce the tensions which contribute to the addictive behaviour and counselling can help patients to deal with the feeling of loss, akin to bereavement, which some people suffer after giving up a pleasurable activity.

Stress management (see Chapter 14)

Suggestions for evaluation and research

- Devise a questionnaire for patients who have new-patient health checks to find out:
  - (a) What the patients expected of the interview.
  - (b) Whether they thought it was beneficial.
  - (c) If they would have liked anything done differently.
- Ask the CPN to accompany you to an appropriate over 75 visit, and compare your assessments of the patient's mental health.
- Review your practice arrangements for well-person screening. Do men and women get comparable services?
- Audit the effectiveness of health promotion activities. What percentage of patients:
  - (a) successfully gave up smoking,
  - (b) reached and maintained a target weight?

References

1. Department of Health (1992) *The Health of the Nation: A Strategy for Health in England*. HMSO, London.
2. (a) Scottish Office (1992) *Scotland's Health – a Challenge to Us All*. HMSO.
    (b) Welsh Office (1992) *Protocols for Investment in Health Gain*. HMSO.
    (c) DHSS (Northern Ireland) (1992) *A Regional Strategy for Northern Ireland*. HMSO.
3. Jones, M. (1993) Working with the new banding; *Primary Health Care*, **3**(7): 4, 6, 8.
4. Larson, E. (1986) Evaluating validity of screening tests; *Nursing Research*, **35**(3): 186–188.
5. Imperial Cancer Research Fund OXCHECK Study Group (1994) Effectiveness of health checks conducted by nurses in primary care: results of the OXCHECK study after one year; *British Medical Journal*, **308**: 308–312.
6. Family Heart Study Group (1994) Randomised controlled trial evaluating cardiovascular screening and intervention in general practice: principal results of the British Family Heart Study; *British Medical Journal*, **308**: 312–320.
7. Cover feature (1993) NHS heal thyself: Health at Work progress report; *Healthlines*, **7**: 12–13.

8. DOH, General Medical Services Committee and RCGP Working Group on Health Promotion (1993) *Better Living – Better Life*. Knowledge House, Henley on Thames.

9. Bower, H. (1993) Seeing health in black and white (using advocates); *Practice Nurse*, **6:** 622.

10. Farooqui, I. (1991) Health promotion and ethnic patients; *The Practitioner*, **235:** 596–599.

11. Hughes, M. (1994) The motivation of Mr 'Yes, but...'; *Practice Nurse*, **7:** 74, 77.

12. Millar, W. and Rollnick, S. (1991) *Motivational Interviewing: Preparing People to Change Addictive Behaviour*. Guildford Press, New York.

13. Lahelma, E. (1992) Unemployment and mental well-being: elaboration of the relationship; *International Journal of Health Services*, **22**(2): 261–274.

14. Basset, C. (1993) Pay attention to the testes; *Practice Nurse*, **5:** 957–58.

15. Garraway, W.M., Russell, E.B., Lee, R.J., Collins, G.N., McKelvie, G.B., Hehir, M., Rogers, A.C. and Simpson, R.J. (1993) Impact of previously unrecognised benign prostatic hypertrophy on daily living activities of middle aged and elderly men; *British Journal of General Practice*, **43,** August: 318–321.

16. Tunstall-Pedoe, H. (1991) The Dundee coronary risk-disk for management of change in risk factors; *British Medical Journal*, **303:** 744–747.

17. Williams, I. (1992) Screening the over 75s; *Practice Nursing*, March: 11.

18. United Kingdom Central Council for Nursing, Midwifery and Health Visiting (1992) *The Scope of Professional Practice*. UKCC, London.

19. Royal College of Nursing (1991) *Assessing Older People: Guidelines for Nurses*. RCN, London.

20. Royal College of Nursing (1993) *Guidelines for Assessing Mental Health Needs in Old Age*. RCN, London.

21. Macintosh, I. (1993) Screening: the hidden costs; *Practice Nursing*, 19 October–1 November: 14.

22. Department of Health (1991) *Health Survey for England*. DOH, London.

23. Ministry of Agriculture, Fisheries and Food, DOH, HEA (1990) *Eight Guidelines for a Healthy Diet*. MAFF, London.

24. Hilgard, E.R., Atkinson, R.C. and Atkinson, R.L. (1971) *Introduction to Psychology* (5th edn). Harcourt Brace Jovanovich, USA.

25. Department of Health (1991) *Dietary Reference Values: A Guide*, HMSO.

26. Jelley, S. (1993) Prescription for health; *Healthlines*, April: 18–19.

27. Hardman, A. (1991) *Exercise and the Heart: Report of a British Heart Foundation Working Group*. British Heart Foundation, London.

28. Barbour, B.G. (1990) Alcohol and pregnancy; *Journal of Nurse-Midwifery*, **35**(2): 78–85.

29. Blackburn, C. and Graham, H. (1993) Information pack – *Smoking among Working Class Mothers*. Department of Applied Social Studies, University of Warwick.

30. DOH, General Medical Services Committee and RCGP Working Group on Health Promotion (1993) *Better Living – Better Life*: 13–14.

Further reading

Jacobs, F. (1994) Ethics in health promotion: freedom or determinism? *British Journal of Nursing*, **3**: 299.

Department of Health (1993) *Targeting Practice: The Contribution of Nurses, Midwives and Health Visitors – The Health of the Nation*. DOH, London.

Teasdale, K.P. (1993) Information and anxiety: a critical reappraisal; *Journal of Advanced Nursing*, **18**: 1125–1132.

Look After Your Heart (1993) *The Health Guide – Helping You to a Healthier Lifestyle*. HEA, London.

Tettersall, M., Sawyer, J. and Salisbury, C. (1991) *Handbook of Practice Nursing*. Churchill Livingstone, Edinburgh.

Useful addresses

Health Education Authority
Hamilton House, Mabledon Place, London WC1H 9TX.

HEA Health Promotion Information Centre
Telephone 071-413 1994/5.

Action on Smoking and Health (ASH)
109 Gloucester Place, London W1H 3PH.
Telephone 071-935 3519.

Smokers Quitline 071-487 3000.
Scottish Smoking Helpline 031-226 5999.

Chapter 10
Child Health and Routine Immunisation

Child health surveillance

The GP Contract allows suitably qualified doctors to be paid for health surveillance of the under fives. In this context 'surveillance' refers to normal growth and development. The purpose of such checks is to detect any problems early, so remedial action can be taken as soon as possible. For example, congenital abnormality of the hip can be corrected in an infant, but permanent disability can result if the condition is not identified in time. Some development checks are performed by the health visitors. The height and weight are recorded on percentile charts, which show where the measurements are in relation to the average for children of the same age and sex (see Appendix 10.1). By using a percentile chart it can be seen when a child's development is falling off in relation to previous records, or to those of his/her peers.

Warning – parents who see the word *surveillance* in records or on the computer screen, can be shocked if they think it means their child is on the 'at-risk' register. A practice nurse may be asked for information, so it can help to be familiar with the specific practice arrangements and to have observed developmental checks being carried out (see Appendix 10.2).

At birth

Every baby has a full medical examination in the neo-natal period. The heart, lungs and eyes are checked, and the weight and head circumference measured. The hips are checked for congenital dislocation (CDH), and the descent of testes is checked in boys. A heel-prick blood test is used to check for congenital hypothyroidism and phenylketonuria; both of which can cause mental retardation if not detected.

6–8 weeks

The GP reviews the pregnancy and family history and discusses any concerns with the parents. A full physical examination, including hips and testes, is carried out and the baby's motor development is tested. The weight, length and head circumference are measured, and the hearing and vision assessed. Normally children show a startle response to a sudden noise or rattle, and can follow a moving object with the eyes to 90° on the horizontal.

8 months

Any parental concerns are discussed and the motor development is assessed. A distraction hearing test is performed, and the eyes are observed for squint or other possible problems with vision.

18 months

The development of language and walking are assessed. A referral is needed for specialised testing at any age if there are any doubts about a child's vision or hearing.

3¹/₂ years

Any parental concerns are discussed and a physical examination carried out as necessary. The height and weight are recorded. Tests are performed of language, gross motor and fine motor development, vision and hearing. The tests are incorporated in activities which are presented as games to the child.

Assessments by the doctor or health visitor are made at other ages as well. All the professional staff should be alert to anything which seems amiss whenever a child is seen in the surgery. A practice nurse might be as concerned about a child which seems unduly passive during a treatment, as about one which wreaks absolute havoc in the treatment room. Teachers and school nurses may report any developmental problems once a child is at school.

Inherited conditions

A child who may have inherited a condition such a sickle cell disease, thalassaemia, or cystic fibrosis may be referred for testing, so that early prophylactic measures can be taken. The rapid growth in the technology may make genetic screening a routine procedure in the not too distant future.

The Royal College of General Practitioners has identified specific areas where intervention may make a dramatic difference to the consequence of a child's development[1]. It is worth everyone bearing these in mind when seeing children at any time:

- contraception (adults)
- encouaging breast-feeding
- discouraging smoking (adults)
- antenatal care
- chemical screening (e.g. phenylketonuria)
- maldescent of the testes (boys)
- childhood immunisation
- hearing
- squint
- visual acuity
- colour vision
- scoliosis
- discouraging smoking (children)
- contraception (children).

A practice nurse's main involvement in child health clinics may consist of giving the immunisations; but sometimes parents will ask for advice or information about other issues. Opportunities for health promotion should not be overlooked.

Health promotion

All adults have a duty to try and prevent accidents and injury to children. Advice can be provided on:

- the safe storage of medicines and chemicals in the home, and the use of child-proof bottle tops and cupboard closing devices,
- potential hazards – stairs, furniture, windows, balconies, cookers, fires, electricity and how to make them safer,
- potentially dangerous toys and games and the risk to health from lack of exercise,
- road safety, safety seats in cars, and protection for cyclists,
- how to avoid personal danger, or get help if abused.

The prevention of coronary heart disease and lifestyle-related illness needs to begin early. Children and adolescents are particularly susceptible to pressure from their peers to experiment with smoking, alcohol, drugs or solvents. A practice nurse can sometimes initiate discussions on these health issues, and be a source of information about the help and services available for worried parents and young people. Joint initiatives with school nurses and health visitors can help to ensure that a consistent message is being put across, and nurses can also act as a pressure group. If hundreds of nurses telephone the TV company to complain every time an actor lights a cigarette in a play on television, it might be more effective in the long run than exhorting young people not to smoke.

Developing sexuality is another major concern for teenagers (see Chapter 12). Nurses with the appropriate training have an important role in promoting sexual health and helping to reduce the number of unwanted pregnancies[2]. The guarantee of confidentiality should encourage more teenagers to seek advice on sexual behaviour and contraception, but many of them are reluctant to visit the surgery; fearing that their parents will be informed[3]. In some areas, community nurses are successfully running services in youth clubs and less formal settings[4].

Child abuse

A practice nurse could be the first to suspect physical or mental abuse to a child. Any abnormal or frequent injuries; particularly those with special significance such as small circular burns (cigarettes?), bruises suggestive of fingertip grasps (upper arms), or from blows (ears and lips). The relationship between the child and parent should also be noted.

The rise in cases of recognised and reported child sexual abuse has highlighted an area in which doctors and nurses have to be particularly vigilant. Any suggestion of sexual abuse, from physical findings, verbal comments or behaviour, must be taken seriously. It is important to deal with these matters confidentially and sensitively. Producing definite evidence is often extremely difficult.

Because of the close relationship with the patients, a practice nurse will be familiar with the background and problems of many local families and be aware of those at risk from factors such as poverty, stress or alcoholism. It should be borne in mind that the incidence of abuse covers all social classes and income groups – not just the socially deprived. Any suspicion of abuse should be discussed with the GP and health visitor.

Every district has a formal child protection policy and staff in general practice must know the procedure to follow. Most health authorities hold regular training on child protection, which practice nurses should attend.

The Children Act 1989

The Children Act gathered all the existing legislation relating to children into a new unified law. Many aspects of the Children Act concern child protection. The need to involve children in decision-making is a key factor[5]. Practice nurses should be aware that any child regardless of age, considered mature enough to understand all the issues, may now give or withhold his/her own consent for treatment.

Childhood immunisation

Organisation

The achievement of immunisation targets involves all the practice team. Payments are only made when a target of 90%, or the lower one of 70% of eligible children is reached. The improved figures for vaccine uptake, since the targets were introduced, make the extra work involved worthwhile.

The current schedule for primary immunisation at two, three and four months of age, consists of diphtheria, tetanus and pertussis vaccine (DTP) given in one injection site, and haemophylus influenzae B injection given in another; plus oral polio drops. Children with definite contraindications to pertussis vaccine should be given diphtheria and tetanus (DT) instead. Inactivated polio vaccine may be given if live virus vaccine is contraindicated for any reason. Mumps, measles and rubella vaccine is given when a child is 12–18 months old, and a pre-school reinforcing dose of diphtheria and tetanus and oral polio is given to children age four to five. Three years should elapse between the third triple injection and the pre-school booster (see Fig. 10.1). From October 1994 a reinforcing injection of low-dose diphtheria toxoid combined with tetanus toxoid (Td) will be given to school leavers with oral polio, instead of tetanus toxoid alone.

Efficient organisation is needed, whether the call/recall system for immunisation is centrally administered or one devised by the individual practice. In some practices the six week developmental check is postponed until the baby is eight weeks old, so that immunisation may be started on the same day. Birthday cards at strategic dates can provide friendly reminders:

- 1 year for MMR
- 4 years for pre-school boosters
- 10 years for rubella (girls who did not have MMR)
- 15 years for tetanus and polio boosters.

Opportunistic immunisation can be aided by 'flagging' the notes of

Age	Vaccine	Dose	Route	
2 months	DTP	0.5 ml	deep sc or im	
	Hib	0.5 ml	deep sc or im	
	Polio	3 drops by mouth		(live vaccine)
3 months	DTP, Hib & Polio as above			
4 months	DTP, Hib & Polio as above			
12–18 months	MMR	0.5 ml	deep sc or im	
4–5 years	DT	0.5 ml	deep sc or im	
	Polio	3 drops by mouth		(live vaccine)
10–11 years	*Rubella	0.5 ml	deep sc or im	(live vaccine)
10–14 years or infancy	BCG	0.1 ml	id	
		0.05 ml	id (<3 months)	
15–19 years	Tetanus	0.5 ml	deep sc or im and	
	Polio	3 drops by mouth		(live vaccine)

Inactive polio vaccine may be used if live vaccine is contraindicated.
* Rubella vaccine is only given routinely to GIRLS who did not receive MMR.

Fig. 10.1 Routine schedule of immunisation.

patients, or those of parents and siblings. Flexible timing of appointments can help, but home visiting may sometimes be necessary.

Any nurse undertaking immunisation needs to be familiar with *Immunisation against Infectious Disease* (the 'Green Book')[6]. This valuable publication is regularly updated and distributed to GP surgeries. It specifies the conditions under which nurses are covered to give immunisations. They are required to work to a protocol and fulfil three criteria:

(1) to be willing to be professionally accountable,
(2) ᴖ have received specific training and be competent in all aspects of immunisation, including contraindications to specific vaccines,
(3) to have had adequate training in dealing with anaphylaxis.

Contraindications to immunisation

Many conditions previously thought to contraindicate immunisation no longer apply. Immunisation should be postponed if the patient has any acute febrile illness. A *severe* local or general reaction to a previous dose would be a definite contraindication to further administration of the same vaccine. Such reactions need to be differentiated from the milder reactions which can often be expected to occur. No child should be denied the protection of immunisation without very good cause.

Live virus vaccines are generally contraindicated for:

- immunosuppressed patients, those receiving high-dose steroids, patients with malignant conditions or other diseases affecting their immune systems,
- pregnant women,
- within three months of receiving immunoglobulin because the immune response may be affected,
- within three weeks of another live vaccine, if not given simultaneously.

The details about specific immunisations and their contraindications are not repeated here, because the 'Green Book' provides such comprehensive information. Access to this book should be one of the standard criteria for immunisation.

The nurse must be sure there are no contraindications to a specific vaccine being given. A medical opinion should be requested when necessary.

Consent

Written consent is preferable as a permanent record. The signed consent should be brought from the parent or legal guardian if anyone else, such as a nanny, brings a child for its injections.

Injection sites

The practice protocol should specify the preferred sites for immunisation, in conjunction with the manufacturer's instructions. The anterolateral aspect of the thigh, the upper arm or upper, outer quadrant of the buttock may be used for DPT and Hib. The upper arm is usually used for older children and adults.

Emergency situations

Anaphylaxis is a rare occurence, but it should always be anticipated. Adrenaline and basic resuscitation equipment must be available. The decision on whether to give immunisations without a doctor being on the premises will depend on the practice policy; plus the individual nurse's experience and willingness to accept the responsibility. Given the potential for tragedy, caution seems sensible. A plan of action for emergencies is essential; especially if giving immunisations in patients' homes.

Information for parents

Written information is useful to reinforce verbal advice about possible reactions and how to deal with them. Infant paracetamol is usually recommended for fever or prolonged crying. Tepid sponging may also be needed for high fever. Parents should know how to get medical help if worried and be asked to report any severe reactions.

DPT vaccine often causes a harmless lump, about the size of a small pea, under the skin. Parents should be told that this can last for several weeks, but will not leave a scar. Any reaction from MMR usually follows the incubation time of the actual diseases. Thus mild syptoms of measles may occur from 7–10 days, possibly with fever and a rash. Mumps takes slightly longer (14–21 days). There may be slight parotid swelling. These reactions are non-infectious, so the children do not need to be isolated.

Other immunisations

Tuberculosis

Bacillus Calmette-Guerin vaccine (BCG) is a live attenuated freeze-dried vaccine not usually available in general practice. In high-risk areas infants may be immunised at birth; otherwise children aged 10–13 receive BCG through the school health service. Some adults may also need immunisation[7]. Parents planning travel to countries with a high incidence of tuberculosis should be advised to consider BCG immunisation for their children[8]. Special training is required to administer BCG vaccine and skin tests. Poor technique can result in unsightly scars.

Special risks

Occasionally immunisation may be needed to protect children at particular risk from contact with hepatitis B, or from influenza or pneumococcal infections which could complicate other medical conditions (see the 'Green Book').

Adult immunisation

The immunisation of adults may be performed for the following reasons:

- missed or incomplete childhood immunisations (vaccines may not have been available then),
- special risk of exposure through injury, occupation, health status, or lifestyle,
- reinforcing doses required to maintain immunity.

Tetanus immunisation

Routine immunisation against tetanus was introduced in 1961, although it was given to people in the armed forces before then. Therefore, patients born before that date, who did not serve in the armed forces, may never have been immunised. They require a primary course of adsorbed tetanus vaccine – three doses of 0.5ml by im or deep sc injection at monthly intervals, and two reinforcing doses at ten yearly intervals. Any unfinished course may be completed at any time without restarting a new course. Once an individual has proof of having received five tetanus injections, boosters are only recommended if a tetanus-prone wound is sustained. Unnecessary booster doses can result in severe local reactions.

A patient with a tetanus-prone wound may require specific antitetanus immunoglobulin in addition to absorbed vaccine, if not fully immunised against tetanus.

Poliomyelitis immunisation

Patients born before 1958 may not have been immunised against polio. Any unimmunised adult should be offered the vaccine. Unless contra-indicated, three doses of oral polio vaccine should be given at monthly intervals. Inactivated vaccine may be used if live virus is contra-indicated. Reinforcing doses are not required, unless at special risk from foreign travel or occupational exposure.

Polio virus can be excreted in the faeces for about six weeks after immunisation. Parents who were not fully immunised themselves should be offered polio vaccine at the same time as their babies, and be warned about careful hand washing after nappy changing.

Rubella immunisation

Hopefully, the immunisation of all children with MMR will eventually remove the main pool of rubella infection. Meanwhile, a new infection risk to pregnant women is emerging – from young males who were too old to be immunised when MMR was first introduced, and who did not contract rubella in childhood; but are succumbing to the disease as adults[9]. All women of child-bearing age should be screened for rubella antibodies and immunised if necessary. A single dose of rubella vaccine 0.5ml by sc or im injection is required. The date of the LMP should be ascertained because rubella immunisation should not be given if pregnancy is a possibility. Women should also be advised not to become pregnant for at least one month after immunisation[8].

Influenza immunisation

Influenza vaccine is produced each year with the three strains of virus likely to be circulating during the winter season. Annual injections of 0.5ml sc or im are required. Patients at particular risk who should be targeted include:

- patients with medical conditions likely to be exacerbated by influenza: diabetes, asthma, chronic respiratory, heart or renal disease,
- immunosuppressed patients,
- residents in institutions where a rapid spread of infection would be likely to occur.

Preparation for the immunisation programme should be made early. Vaccines can be bought in bulk from the manufacturer, if suitable storage is available. A small profit can be made this way. Prescriptions have to be issued for each injection given, saved carefully and sent to the Prescription Pricing Authority once a month. Alternatively, individual patients are issued with a prescription for the vaccine, which they get from the chemist and return for the injection. Patients at risk can be identified from disease and age/sex registers. Special 'flu jab' clinics may be set up and invitations sent out. The best time to start the programme is mid-October. That way the bulk of the injections will be completed before the end of the year to protect patients early in the following year when influenza epidemics are most likely.

Contraindications to influenza vaccine include:

- any febrile illness (postpone injection until recovered),
- severe adverse reaction to a previous dose,
- hypersensitivity to egg (previous anaphylactic reaction),
- pregnancy.

Adverse reactions are usually mild. Soreness may occur at the injection site. Fever, malaise, myalgia may occur a few hours after immunisation and last up to two days. Rarely there might be allergic reactions if the patient is hypersensitive to egg protein because the virus is cultured in eggs to produce the vaccine.

Pneumococcal immunisation

An encapsulated strain of *Streptococcus pneumoniae* can cause pneumonia, bacteraemia or meningitis. Susceptible patients who should be offered immunisation include people with:

- chronic lung, heart, liver or renal conditions,
- disorders of immunity through disease or treatment,
- diabetes mellitus,
- disease of spleen or splenectomy,
- homozygous sickle cell disease.

A single dose of pneumovax 0.5ml sc or im is required. It may be given at the same time as a 'flu jab', but at a different injection site.

Specific contraindication – reimmunisation within three years of receiving pneumococcal immunisation.

Adverse reactions – mild soreness at injection site and slight fever.

Hepatitis B

This highly infectious virus is spread by blood contact through contaminated sharps or needles, sexual intercourse, mother to child at birth, or a bite from an infected person.

Active immunisation

Immunisation is recommended for people at particular risk:

- health care personnel,
- patient contacts from haemodylysis, haematology or oncology departments,
- plasma fraction workers,
- drug abusers,
- patients at increased risk due to sexual activities (some homosexual men),
- travellers going to reside in areas where hepatitis B is endemic,
- close contacts with patients with hepatitis B, or healthy carriers of the virus.

The hepatitis B vaccine is prepared from yeast cells. Three intramuscular doses of 1ml are required for adults; the second dose one month, and the third, six months after the initial injection. (0.5ml for children 0–12 years). Injection should be into the deltoid muscle instead of the buttock. (The anterolateral thigh should be used for infants). Patients with haemophilia, when injection could cause bleeding into the muscle, may be given subcutaneous or intradermal injection at the discretion of the GP.

Antibody levels should be checked about six months after the completion of the course. Further doses are sometimes required to achieve immunity. Reinforcing doses may be required after five years.

Adverse reactions include redness and soreness at the injection site. More rarely – fever, rash, flu-like symptoms, arthralgia and/or abnormal liver function tests.

Passive immunisation

Hepatitis B immunoglobulin may be required for anyone at immediate risk after exposure to the disease. Active immunisation should be started simultaneously with an injection of hepatitis B vaccine given at a different injection site.

Hepatitis A

Protection against hepatitis A is usually required for travellers. However, now that active immunisation is possible it should be considered for occupational groups at particular risk – for example sewerage workers. Carers and residents in institutions where outbreaks of hepatitis A are likely may also be considered for immunisation. Three injections are required for lasting immunity – 1ml im into the deltoid muscle, repeated after 2–4 weeks and 6–12 months.

Immunoglobulin may be used for short-term protection for people in close contact with the disease.

Conclusion

Achieving a high uptake of immunisation makes a worthwhile contribution to the health of the population. Practice nurses now provide a wide range of vaccines, but time also needs to be made available when planning appointments, to help educate the public about the cause, means of spread and hygiene measures needed to prevent the transmission of infectious diseases. This is particularly important because the success of immunisation means that many people will never have seen the effects of those diseases.

Suggestions for evaluation and research

- Review the service provided for young people by your practice:
    (a) What information is available specifically for them?
    (b) How easy is it for children under 16 to make their own appointments if they wish to do so?
    (c) Do all the medical and nursing staff understand the law relating to contraception for girls under 16?
    (d) Is everyone in the practice familiar with the district child protection policy?
- Conduct a study of one aspect of teenage health relevant to your practice population. Discuss with the health visitor how the issue might be tackled within the practice.
- Audit the incidence and severity of any reactions after immunisation to see if:
    (a) The injection technique could be improved or altered.
    (b) The patients/parents were given appropriate information about possible side-effects.
- Compile a disease register of all the patients who have had a splenectomy. Have they been offered pneumococcal vaccine?

References

1. Royal College of General Practitioners (1988) *Healthier Children – Thinking Prevention: report of a working party appointed by the Royal College of General Practitioners*, (3rd Edn). RCGP, London.
2. Cook, R. (1993) Preventing unwanted teenage pregnancies; *Nursing Standard*, **7**(38): 28–30.
3. Scally, G. (1993) Confidentiality, contraception and young people; *British Medical Journal*, **307**: 1157–1158.
4. Cassidy, J. (1994) Sex and drugs and rock 'n' roll; *Nursing Times*, **90**(1): 14–15.
5. Department of Health (1992) *The Children Act 1989 – What every Nurse, Health Visitor and Midwife should know*; DOH Health Publications Unit.
6. DOH, Welsh Office, Scottish Office Home and Health Department, DHSS (Northern Ireland) (1992) *Immunisation against Infectious Disease*. HMSO, London.
7. Watson, J.M. (1993) TB in Britain today; *British Medical Journal* **306:** 221–222.

8. Mitchinson, D.A. and Ellis, C. in Dawood, R. (Ed.) (1992) *Travellers' Health – How to Stay Healthy Abroad* (3rd Edn): 80–82. Oxford University Press, Oxford.
9. Wise, J. (1993) Sixfold rise in rubella cases leads to alarm; *MIMS Magazine Weekly*, 9 March: 2.

Further reading

Sheridan, M. (1975) *From Birth to Five Years – Children's Developmental Progress* (3rd Edn). Routledge, London.
Hall, D.M.B. (Ed.) (1989) *Health for all Children: a Programme for Child Health Surveillance*. Oxford University Press, Oxford.
Hall, D.M.B., Hill, P. and Elliman, D. (1990) *The Child Health Surveillance Handbook*. Radcliffe Medical Press, Oxford.
NHS Management Executive (1993) *Sickle Cell Anaemia*. DOH Information Office, Leeds.

Useful addresses

Brook Advisory Centres
153a East Street, London SE17 2SD.
Telephone 071-708 1234.
Write or phone for details of centres in other cities. Brook Helpline 071-410 0420 (24-hour recorded information).

Appendix 10.1
Example of a percentile chart

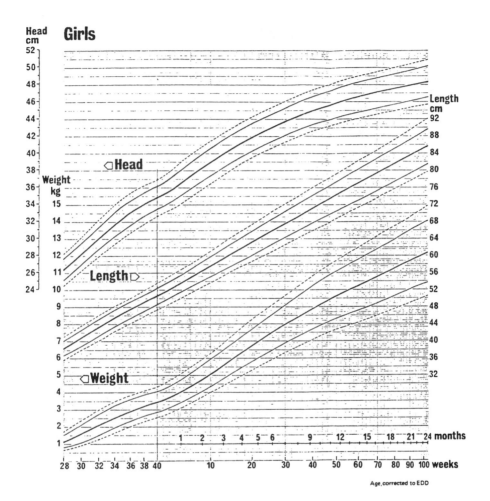

Age,corrected to EDD

Appendix 10.2
Example of a developmental assessment chart

DEVELOPMENT CHART   (GM = Gross motor: FM = Fine motor: S = Social: L = Language)

1. Mark "X" for items which child could perform.
2. Mark "O" for items which child could not perform.
3. For items which could not be, or were not tested enter "N.T." instead of "X" or "O".
4. The rectangles give the expected abilities at each age. Where an expected function is not achieved, test abilities higher up the same vertical column.
5. Record Mother's observations and results of Physical Examination in right hand column.
6. Summary: "N" = Normal. "O" = Requires Observation. "AB" = Abnormal, requiring investigation.

		Actual Age	6 / 52	3 / 12	6 / 12	9 / 12	12 / 12	18 / 12	2 yr.	3 yr.	4 yr.	Physical Examination; Mother's Comments	N	O	AB	
6 weeks	GM	Lifted prone, momentarily holds head in line with body.														DOCTOR
		Lies prone with pelvis flat, hips extended.														
		Pull to sit, head lag partly controlled														
	FM	Hands closed														
		Grasp reflex +														
	S	Smiles at mother														
		Follows objects side to middle														
	L	Single vowels, ah, eh, uh.										Hips				
3 months	GM	Lifted prone, holds head up														DR. OR NURSE
		Lying prone lifts head 45° – 90°														
		Pull to sit – only slight head lag														
	FM	Hands loosely open														
		Holds rattle momentarily.														
	S	Supine, watches own hands														
		Follows objects side to side														
	L	Squeals of pleasure														
6 months	GM	Lying prone, back is extended and weight on hands (not arms)														DR. OR NURSE
		Rolls prone to supine														
		Sits up with hands forward for support														
		Weight bearing on legs														
	FM	Cubes grasped against thenar eminence														
		Transfers cubes from one hand to other														
		Reaches out for objects														
	S	Alert: responds to mother and examiner										Hips				
	L	Smiles and laughs														
		Gurgles and coos														

P.K.U. — Blood phenylanine

SUMMARY

DOCTOR | DR. OR NURSE | DR. OR NURSE | DOCTOR

9 months

- GM: Sits steadily / Stands up, holding on / Creeps on hands and knees
- FM: Crude thumb-finger grasp
- S: Waves "bye-bye" / Knows his own name
- L: Hearing Responses at 18" (Lt. and Rt.) — Prompt | Delayed | Nil

Cup and Spoon
Rattle
"OOO"
"PSS"

Visual Acuity (Sycar Balls)

12 months

- GM: Pivots stably while sitting / Walks — one hand held
- FM: Fine pincer grasp — finger/thumb / Throws objects down and watches
- S: Plays "Peep-bo" / Responds to simple commands / Uses 2 - 3 words with meaning
- L: Throws ball without falling

Squint

18 months

- GM: Walks upstairs, one hand held / Builds 3 - 4 cubes
- FM: Feeds without rotating spoon / Dry by day mostly
- S: Understands simple orders / Several intelligible words

Hips

2 years

- GM: Kicks ball without overbalancing / Walks backward in imitation
- FM: Unscrews lids, turns door knobs / Builds 6 - 7 cubes / Can put on shoes and socks
- S: Watches others play, but does not join in / Asks for drink, food, toilet
- L: Joins 2 or 3 words in sentences

Hearing Responses at 4' (Lt. and Rt.) — Prompt | Delayed | Nil

Simple commands
Name spoken
?'s with pictures

Visual Acuity (Sycar Toys)

Squint

	DR. OR NURSE	DOCTOR	DOCTOR

3 years

GM
- Can stand on one foot
- Jumps off bottom step

FM
- Builds 9 cubes
- Can dress fully except for buttons
- Draws man on request

S
- Joins in play

L
- Constantly asking questions

4 years

GM
- Hops on one foot
- Can button clothes fully

FM
- Attends to own toilet needs
- Imaginative play

S
- Tells stories

L
- Counts up to Ten
- Questioning at its height

Hearing Responses at 4' (Lt. and Rt.)

	Prompt	Delayed	Nil
Simple commands			
Questions with picture book			

Visual Acuity

Lt.   Rt.

Squint

PRESCHOOL ASSESSMENT AND SUMMARY

Chapter 11
Travel Health

Business in Thailand, honeymoons in India, or long weekends in the Gambia – nothing is impossible nowadays. However, that also means more people are at risk of contracting unpleasant diseases, and immunisation alone does not give sufficient protection. Backpackers can face particular hazards when travelling rough. Above all, travellers need information about the risks, preventive measures, and what do if illness occurs. Many practice nurses are accepting this responsibility, which by its complexity, calls for high standards of care. The nurse should have an agreed immunisation protocol, adequate knowledge, and access to suitable reference material.

Nurse education

Travel health is invariably covered on practice nurse courses. More specialist training is available at travel clinics, such as the clinic at the London Hospital for Tropical Diseases. Study days are run regularly by local practice nurse groups, facilitators, vaccine companies, and nursing journals.

Resources

- A computerised system gives regular updates via a modem link, to the Medical Advisory Services for Travellers Abroad (MASTA).
- Information on disease risks and immunisation is published monthly in *Pulse*, *MIMS* and other journals.
- Local communicable disease department (often linked to TRAVAX).
- Telephone information services run by the Evans and Merieux vaccine companies provide information about health risks and advice about immunisation.
- *Immunisation against Infectious Diseases* (the 'Green Book'[1]) and *International Travel and Health* (the 'Yellow Book'[2]) should be standard reference books.

- *Travellers' Health – How to Stay Healthy Abroad*[3], is packed with information on all aspects of travel health.
- The Department of Health's leaflet *Health Advice for Travellers*, can be obtained in bulk for distribution to patients. The leaflets are updated regularly, so avoid stock-piling out-of-date ones. Leaflets are available from the same source on avoiding hepatitis B and HIV infection abroad[4].

It is helpful if patients fill in a form outlining their travel plans and immunisation status, so that advice can be tailored to their needs. Specialist help may be needed with complicated itineraries. 'MASTA' will provide written health briefs for individual patients, so it is useful to keep a stock of application forms.

Food and water

Diarrhoea is one of the most common problems for travellers. Detailed advice on hand washing and food and water safety may prevent a journey from becoming a disaster. Bacteria multiply more quickly in hot climates so extra special care is needed where hygiene standards are suspect:

Advice	Rationale
Eat only freshly prepared and cooked hot food.	Before bacterial growth can occur in food.
Avoid salads, and choose fruit and vegetables that can be peeled.	Human excreta may be used as a fertiliser.
Avoid shellfish.	Feeding method concentrates micro-organisms.
Avoid raw meat and fish.	Worm infestation risk.
Boil or avoid unpasteurised milk. Avoid suspect ice-cream	Risk of tuberculosis and brucellosis etc.
Boil or sterilise unsafe water or use bottled water. Check the seal on all bottles.	May be contaminated with human or animal excreta. Make sure bottle has not been filled from a tap!
Avoid ice in drinks. Use 'safe' water for cleaning teeth.	Even small amounts of unsafe water can be hazardous.
Recreational water may be unsafe.	Pools may be contaminated if not well-chlorinated. Bilharzia risk from some freshwater[5].

Diarrhoea advice

If diarrhoea does occur most cases will resolve within two to three days. Whatever the cause, dehydration is the major complication, so fluid replacement is essential. Mildly affected healthy adults may only need plenty of non-alcoholic drinks; but in all other cases, rehydration fluid should be used. Use commercially produced sachets, or make up a solution with four heaped teaspoonsful of sugar or honey and one level teaspoonful of salt in one litre of 'safe' water. Continue with small, regular amounts even if vomiting occurs. Seek medical help for very young children, elderly or frail people, those with other medical conditions like diabetes, or if diarrhoea contains blood or the patient becomes more ill.

Antidiarrhoea medication may delay infection being flushed from the body, so use only when toilet facilities are unavailable, e.g. on long bus journeys. Do not use if blood in the diarrhoea occurs[7].

Remember that diarrhoea can make the contraceptive pill ineffective because it passes through the gut without the time to be absorbed.

Malaria

Female *Anopheles* mosquitos transmit the parasites that cause malaria in their saliva. Protection against bites is often more important than drug prophylaxis because drug resistance is becoming such a serious problem. Of the four species of malaria parasites, *plasmodium falciparum* is the most serious – causing death in about 1% of travellers infected. Up-to-date information on anti-malarial drugs can be obtained from the Malaria Reference Laboratory. Travellers at risk on long trips to remote places should have drugs and information for treating malaria, in case infection does occur (see *MIMS*). People who once lived in a malarious area must be warned of their particular risk when returning, as they may have lost their previous immunity but fail to take adequate precautions against mosquito bites. Advice on malaria should cover the following points:

- *Personal protection.* Try to avoid being bitten. Keep arms, legs and feet covered after sunset because mosquitoes feed after dusk. Use insect repellents containing diethyl tolumide (deet), or similar chemicals, to deter biting. These may be applied to the skin with caution, or clothes can be impregnated with deet for a more lasting effect. Impregnated wrist and ankle bands may also be helpful.
- *Protection at night.* If using air conditioning, make sure that windows and doors are closed properly and use an insecticide spray.

If mosquitoes are able to enter at night use a mosquito net. Make sure it is has no holes or tears and tuck it properly under the mattress. Mosquitoes will bite through a net if the sleeper's body is in contact with it. Nets impregnated with permethrin will kill or repel mosquitoes, so are more effective. Mosquito coils or electrically operated vapourisers may also be of use – providing they last until daybreak. Electricity supplies are often unreliable.

- *Anti-malarial tablets.* These do not prevent infection from occurring. Their main effect is on the the parasites' life cycle after the liver stage. Hence the need to continue taking tablets for at least four weeks after leaving the risk area. Tablets should be started one week before arrival, to ensure an adequate level of drug in the bloodstream, and taken religiously while there. Patients should be warned about possible side-effects (see *MIMS*). Mefloquine (*Larium*) must not be given to women if there is any likelihood of pregnancy within three months of taking them. It is also contraindicated for patients with epilepsy or a history of psychiatric disturbance.
- *If unwell, or a fever develops.* Medical help should be sought within 24 hours. Early treatment of malaria can prevent a fatal outcome. If illness occurs after returning home, the doctor should be told about the trip abroad[7].

The degree of risk from malaria needs to be ascertained and the appropriate prophylaxis advised. Charts are published monthly in *Pulse*, *MIMS* and other journals, giving the recommended anti-malarial regimes. Chloroquine and proguanil can be purchased in a pharmacy. A private prescription is required for mefloquine. All the tablets can cause nausea and gastric disturbance. Patients should be advised to take them after the evening meal because the effects may not be noticed so much during the night.

Sun exposure

Patients should be warned about the risks of exposure to too much sun. Long-term exposure can cause skin cancer; especially as the ozone layer which filters out dangerous ultraviolet radiation is being destroyed. Sunburn may ruin a holiday, and in extreme cases could be fatal. Falling asleep in the sun is a big danger. Generally speaking, the fairer the skin, the greater the risk of burning. Children need special vigilance and protection from the sun.

Sensible precautions for sunbathers should include gradual acclimatisation (beginning with only 10–15 minutes a day), and the regular application of sunscreens. Reapplication will be needed after swimming or showering.

Water, sand and snow will all increase the reflection of ultraviolet, so extra care is needed to protect skin on beaches, ski-slopes or when taking part in water sports. A moisturising cream should be applied after exposure to the sun and regular drinks are needed to replace fluid loss. Alcohol causes dehydration and should therefore be limited. If urine is dark and concentrated – more fluids are needed. Salt lost in sweat will also need replacing – either in the diet, or if excessive sweating, by also adding half a level teaspoonful of salt per litre of liquid for drinking. Severe sunburn will need medical treatment[8].

Heatstroke

Heatstroke may happen without direct exposure to the sun. Impairment of the heat-regulating system causes a dangerous rise in body temperature as sweating diminishes. Death can occur within a few hours if not treated. Immediate cooling by evaporation is needed, using wet sheets or towels on the skin and fanning. Rehydration with cool drinks is also essential, and emergency medical treatment should be obtained. Patients should be warned of the contributing factors to heatstroke, especially for anyone with a skin condition which impairs sweating:

- continuous overheating
- being overweight and unfit
- alcohol excess
- physical exertion
- unsuitable clothing
- some drugs, including cold cures and diuretics[9].

Hepatitis B and HIV infections

The holiday atmosphere and alcohol may combine to remove inhibitions, but may also result in unwanted souvenirs. Casual sexual encounters lead to the spread of sexually transmitted diseases (including HBV and HIV). The prostitutes in many countries could be infected, and patients should be warned of the serious risks. If used correctly, condoms provide a degree of protection, but they should be stored in a cool place away from direct sunlight, and particular care is needed to prevent their being damaged in transit.

Intravenous drug users are liable to contract HIV and hepatitis B infection through sharing needles. The obvious advice is not to inject, or not to share equipment. Tattooing, acupuncture, and ear piercing should also be avoided. Emergency medical or dental treatment may expose travellers to risk in countries where the re-use of equipment is likely. Sterile emergency packs containing syringes, needles, sutures and blood transfusion needles can be purchased for a reasonable price, but blood transfusion should be avoided if at all possible in high risk countries. Travellers should be advised to have sufficient health insurance to be flown home in an emergency.

High altitude

The reduced atmospheric pressure at high altitudes means that less oxygen is available to the tissues. The body adapts by deeper respirations and a faster heart rate, but time for acclimatisation is necessary and fatalities do occur. Patients planning journeys to high altitudes should seek medical advice; especially if they have respiratory or cardiac conditions.

Air travel

Flying at high altitude, despite cabin pressurisation, may also cause problems of hypoxia for some people; particularly those who smoke heavily[10]. The ears are likely to be affected by changes in air pressure, and severe discomfort may be caused if congestion blocks the eustachian tubes. Patients with medical problems should ask a doctor to check their fitness to fly. The venous return can be slowed when sitting in a cramped seat for long periods and can cause a deep vein thrombosis. Therefore the importance of regular movement and ankle exercises should be explained.

Travel in pregnancy

Pregnant women should be advised not to travel to remote areas, but if such travel is essential, then between 18 and 24 weeks gestation are considered to be the most suitable times[11]. Air travel in normal pregnancy is generally considered safe up to 32 weeks, but women should check with their particular airline. A doctor's letter may be required, and adequate health insurance is essential.

Immunisation should be avoided in pregnancy – except when the risk from the disease outweighs the risk from the vaccine.

Travel for patients with diabetes

Patients with diabetes should obtain advice before long journeys – especially if crossing time zones. The points to be considered are as follows.

- Carry a letter from a medical practitioner about the diabetes and the need for injections (if applicable).
- Carry emergency carbohydrates in the hand-luggage.
- Carry all the insulin in the hand-luggage (in case baggage gets mislaid, and because the insulin might freeze in the hold if travelling by air). If not travelling alone get a companion to carry spare insulin and equipment (in case of mishaps). Use an insulated bag to keep the insulin cool.
- Take medication, if needed, to prevent travel sickness.
- Follow the normal sickness advice if vomiting or diarrhoea occur (see Chapter 15 *Appendix 15.1*).
- Make sure the travel insurance is adequate, and that the insurer knows about the diabetes[12].

Travel for patients with asthma (see Chapter 15)

Patients who have asthma should be advised to plan holidays and business trips carefully and know what to do in an emergency. Points to be considered include:

- Ensure an adequate supply of 'preventer' and 'reliever' drugs, including spares in case of loss or damage.
- Ensure that the delivery systems is appropriate, dry powder capsules may deteriorate in very hot and humid conditions.
- Make sure the patient knows how to recognise the signs of deteriorating asthma control, and knows what action to take. A course of oral steroids, and possibly antibiotics, may be prescribed for emergency use.
- A doctor's letter may be a good idea – outlining the condition and treatment.
- A portable nebuliser or large volume spacer may be carried for routine or emergency use.
- Trips should be planned where possible to avoid known trigger factors e.g. grass pollen, animals or cold air.
- Make sure there is suitable travel health insurance.
- Make a note of local medical facilities and telephone numbers after arriving at the destination.

The National Asthma Campaign booklet – *The Asthmatic on Holiday* gives useful advice on planning suitable holidays.

Immunisation for travellers

Practice nurses often work out schedules of immunisation for travellers; however the doctor is responsible for prescribing vaccines, so the protocol should specify the arrangements to be adopted. Many surgeries now purchase the vaccines and claim reimbursement and dispensing fees. The bulk storage of vaccines needs special care and temperature control (see Chapter 5).

Immunisation serves two purposes: to prevent the spread of disease, and to protect the individual from infection. Proof of immunisation may be mandatory in some countries, and entry can be denied without a valid certificate of immunisation. Yellow fever is the only disease for which an International Certificate of Immunisation may still be required. Cholera certificates are still demanded in some countries; although the current vaccine has doubtful value, and is no longer recommended by the World Health Organisation[13]. Travellers to Saudi Arabia require proof of meningitis immunisation.

Individual schedules of immunisation will depend on:

- The injections previously received.
- The length and type of journey.
- The time available before departure.

Accelerated schedules are possible, but it is best to start six to eight weeks before departure (14 weeks if a full course of tetanus and/or polio is needed). Some diseases are seasonal, so up-to-date information is necessary. The travel charts in *Pulse, MIMS* etc., are suitable for straightforward trips. The telephone information services, and MASTA will advise on more complicated journeys. The 'Green Book' gives essential information about all the vaccines, doses, contraindications and side-effects. The safeguards and emergency procedures should be specified in the protocol (see Chapter 5 *Injections*).

All the vaccines administered, and specific advice given, must be recorded accurately in the patient's records. Computer records of immunisation save time when planning future schedules, and are valuable for administration and audit purposes too.

Item of service fees may be claimed for most immunisations on FP73 claim forms supplied by the FHSA. Fees for temporary residents cannot be claimed as well as item of service fees if immunisations only are given; but both are allowed if travel health or other medical advice is given as well[14].

Contraindications

A check list helps to ensure that no essential questions are omitted:

Questions	Rationale
Are you well today? If NO, what is the problem?	Postpone immunisation if acute or febrile illness.
Are you taking steroids? Are you having treatment, or have you any condition which affects your immune system?	Live viruses should not be given to immunosuppressed patients. Medical advice needed before any vaccines given, if any doubts exist.
Is there any chance that you might be pregnant? (Female patients.)	Vaccines should not be administered unless risk of disease outweighs possible risk to the foetus.
Have you reacted badly to any previous vaccine?	Risk of anaphylaxis, or serious reaction if allergic.
Are you allergic to eggs or any medicines?	Previous anaphylactic reaction to eggs contraindicates yellow fever immunisation.
	Some vaccines contain traces of antibiotics.

The manufacturers' instructions for administration and contra-indications to immunisation must always be observed.

Tetanus

This risk occurs throughout the world. A primary course or booster is recommended for anyone not already protected.

Polio

This is still prevalent in many developing countries. A primary course or booster is recommended for anyone travelling outside northern Europe, Australia, New Zealand or North America, who is not fully immunised.

Typhoid

This is a salmonella infection transmitted by food or drink contaminated by the excreta of a person suffering from the disease, or from a healthy carrier. The food and drink precautions given above are as important as the immunisation. Three types of typhoid vaccines are available:

(1) *Heat-killed, phenol-preserved monovalent vaccine.* The primary course consists of two doses four to six weeks apart. Reinforcing doses can be given after three years, if needed. The vaccine often causes severe flu-like symptoms and a very painful arm after the injection. Second and subsequent injections can be given intra-dermally, but many practices now use the newer vaccines which cause less discomfort.
(2) *Vi capsular polysaccharide vaccine (Typhim Vi).* One dose gives protection for three years and causes less severe reactions around the injection site, and only mild systemic effects. The single dose is easier to fit into immunisation schedules.
(3) *Attenuated live oral vaccine (Vivotif).* This is a live oral vaccine consisting of three capsules; one to be taken alternate daily. Three capsules give protection for three years, but the instructions for storing the capsules and timing the doses must be followed. It is not recommended for children under six years old.

Hepatitis A

This is caused by faecal contamination of food and water. The disease is usually mild in young children and may not be recognised[15]. Active immunisation is now possible with Havrix for adults, and the newer vaccine, Havrix Junior, which can be given to children age 1–15 years. Three doses give protection for up to ten years. The vaccine is expensive, so patients must be encouraged to complete the course, in order to make it cost-effective. Ideally, blood should be taken beforehand to test for hepatitis antibodies, as many adults will already be immune.

Havrix is suitable for regular travellers and those planning to live in places where exposure to the infection is likely. Passive immunity may be provided by *normal human immunoglobulin (HNIG)* for infrequent, short-term visits.

Patients should be made aware that this is a blood product, even though there is no known risk of contracting any infection from it. HNIG may affect the development of immunity from live virus vaccines, although yellow fever vaccine is generally unaffected in the UK because HNIG does not usually contain antibody to this virus. Oral polio and other live virus vaccines should be given at least three weeks before or three months after immunoglobulin. They may be given on the same day in accelerated schedules of immunisation.

Hepatitis B

Immunisation is not routinely recommended as a travel vaccine. However, it may sometimes be offered to people planning to spend long periods abroad and to travellers such as health workers, likely to be at special risk.

Yellow fever

This is a viral infection transmitted by mosquito bites in tropical Africa and South America. The incubation period is three to six days. Immunisation is given only at designated centres, but with the increase in foreign travel, many practices have now been accepted as yellow fever centres by the Department of Health. The 'Green Book' contains a list of the designated centres.

An International Certificate of Immunisation is issued after immunisation. One dose conveys immunity for ten years, so patients should be advised to take care of their certificates during that time. A private fee can be charged because the vaccine has to be purchased and is not reimbursable.

Meningococcal meningitis

This disease usually occurs in epidemics. It is spread by droplets, so is most common in areas where people are crowded together. Visitors to the 'meningitis belt of Africa', northern India, and the lowlands of Nepal during the dry seasons may be at risk of meningitis. Visitors to the Hajj in Mecca without a certificate of meningitis immunisation will be denied entry to Saudi Arabia. The vaccine must have been given not more than three years ago, or less than ten days for the certificate to be valid. One dose of Meningitis A and C vaccine provides immunity for three years for adults and children over two months of age.

Rabies

This is a viral infection, usually transmitted by the bite of an infected animal. Pre-exposure immunisation may be offered to travellers to remote areas where they may be more than 24 hours journey time away from a hospital. A course of three injections provides some protection for up to three years. The vaccine is usually prescribed on a private prescription. Post-exposure treatment is still needed if bitten. A patient who is scratched or bitten by an animal which could have rabies should also be advised:

- to cleanse the wound thoroughly with soap and water,
- to get the name and address of the animal's owner (if known), so the animal can be observed for signs of rabies,
- to get advice from a local doctor about the risk of rabies in that area.

Japanese B encephalitis

A viral disease spread by mosquitoes, is most commonly found in rural Asian countries during the monsoon season, where there are concentrations of animals near rice fields. People travelling rough are most at risk. An inactivated vaccine is available on a named-patient basis only, usually by private prescription.

Tick borne encephalitis

This is caused by a virus transmitted by the bite of an infected animal tick; mainly during the spring and summer. Ticks are picked up from the undergrowth in warm, forested areas of Europe and Scandinavia. Hikers and campers are most at risk. People planning trips to those areas are advised not to walk with bare legs and to use an insect repellent. A killed vaccine is available on a named-patient basis. A full course to last three years requires three injections. Two injections give protection for one year.

Suggestions for evaluation and research

- Review all the travel health reference material available to the nurses and patients in the practice. Is it up-to-date?
- Review the appointment times. Are the consultation times long enough to cover all the necessary aspects of travel health?
- Devise a questionnaire to find out what health risks patients perceive from travel to Africa, Asia or South America:
    (a) How aware are the patients of the major health risks?
    (b) How could your travel health promotion be improved?
- Devise a study of the advantages and disadvantages of using the newer travel vaccines. What are the cost implications?
- Audit the number of patients who are treated for illness on return from abroad? How many of them had been given specific travel health advice?

References

1. DOH, Welsh Office, Scottish Office Home and Health Department, DHSS (Northern Ireland) (1992) *Immunisation against Infectious Disease.* HMSO, London.
2. World Health Organisation (1993) *International Travel and Health – Vaccination Requirements and Health Advice.* HMSO, London.
3. Dawood, R. (Ed.) (1992) *Travellers' Health – How to stay Healthy Abroad* (3rd Edn). Oxford University Press, Oxford.
4. Department of Health (1993) *Avoiding the Risk of HIV for Travellers – Travelsafe advice from the Department of Health.* Health Distribution Unit, Heywood.
5. Dawood, R. (Ed.) (1992) *Travellers' Health – How to Stay Healthy Abroad*; Appendix 5. OUP, Oxford.
6. Barer, M. and Behrens, R. In: Dawood, R. Ed. (1992) *Travellers' Health – How to Stay Healthy Abroad*: 15–32. OUP, Oxford.
7. Hall, A.P. In: Dawood, R. Ed. (1992) *Travellers' Health – How to Stay Healthy Abroad*: 103–113. OUP, Oxford.
8. Hawk, J.L.A. In: Dawood, R. Ed. (1992) *Travellers' Health – How to Stay Healthy Abroad*: 249–255. OUP, Oxford.
9. Adam, J.M. In: Dawood, R. Ed. (1992) *Travellers' Health – How to Stay Healthy Abroad*: 237–238. OUP, Oxford.
10. Harding, R. In: Dawood, R. Ed. (1992) *Travellers' Health – How to Stay Healthy Abroad*: 188. OUP, Oxford.
11. Brant, H.A. In: Dawood, R. Ed. (1992) *Travellers' Health – How to Stay Healthy Abroad*: 336–340. OUP, Oxford.
12. Watkins, P. In: Dawood, R. Ed. (1992) *Travellers' Health – How to Stay Healthy Abroad*: 353–358. OUP, Oxford.
13. DOH, Welsh Office, Scottish Home and Health Department, DHSS (Northern Ireland) (1992) *Immunisation against Infectious Disease*: 131. HMSO, London.
14. DOH, Welsh Office *Statement of Fees and Allowances to General Medical Practitioners in England and Wales from 1990*: paragraph 32.12.
15. Waterson, T. In: Dawood, R. (Ed.) (1992) *Travellers' Health – How to Stay Healthy Abroad* (3rd Edn): 349. OUP, Oxford.

Further reading

Turner, A.C. (1991) *The Traveller's Health Guide* (4th Edn). Lascelles.

Useful addresses

Medical Advisory Service for Travellers Abroad (MASTA)
London School of Hygiene and Tropical Medicine,
Keppel Street, London WC1E 7BR.
Telephone 071-831 5333 for information about local travel clinics.
071-631 4408 (*Fax* 071-436 5389) for printed health advice about individual travel itineries; a fee is charged.
MASTA Healthline 0891-224100 (computerised tape service for free health briefs).

Malaria Reference Laboratory
London School of Hygiene and Tropical Medicine
Telephone 071-927 2212 (recorded information).

Hospital for Tropical Diseases
4 St Pancras Way, London NW1 0PE.
Telephone 071-387 4411.
Healthline (recorded information) 0839-337733.

Liverpool School of Tropical Medicine
Pembroke Place, Liverpool L3 5QA.
Telephone 051-708 9393.

Communicable Diseases Unit
Ruchill Hospital, Glasgow G20 9NB
Telephone 041-946 7120.

Central Public Health Laboratory
61 Colindale Avenue, London NW9 5EQ.
Telephone 081-200 4400.

Merieux Vaccination Information Service
Telephone 0628-773737.

Evans Vaccination Information Service
Telephone 0625-537607.

Department of Health information leaflets
BAPS, Health Distribution Unit,
Heywood Stores, Lancs OL10 2PZ

Chapter 12
Sexual Health

When a practice provides a comprehensive range of services, the patients have the added advantage of continuity of care. Targets in the *Health of the Nation* strategy include a reduction in sexually transmitted diseases, and a reduction in conception by girls under 16. Primary health care workers need to pay more attention to sexual health issues if the targets are to be met. Practice nurses see patients of all ages and have the opportunity to promote sexual health as a part of healthy living. There are several aspects to sexual health:

- having a positive sense of sexual identity and self-worth,
- being able to sustain mutually satisfying relationships in which both partners feel secure enough to express personal needs or wishes,
- preventing unwanted pregnancies,
- avoiding sexually transmitted diseases.

Sexual identity

Sexual identity involves more than male or female gender, (which is usually decided *in utero*). Biologically there is little difference between the male and female sexual response[1], but social influences play a major part in the development of sexuality[2]. Practice nurses need to be aware of cultural differences and the variety of ways in which sexuality can be expressed. Ideas of masculinity and femininity undergo periodic changes. In areas of high male unemployment many men who previously had a dominant role in the household lose their sense of self-worth as their wives find employment instead. In other areas women expect equality with men as a right, but this change in the balance of power can cause conflict. For example, some women can be frustrated in their attempts to achieve their full potential, while some men are made to feel inadequate by assertive females. Conflict can occur in Asian families, for example, when young people brought up in the West rebel against arranged marriages, dress codes, or male domination.

In a predominantly heterosexual society, minority groups are having to campaign for equality. Attitudes to homosexuality are gradually changing, but a great deal of homophobia still exists. Anybody who feels uncomfortable dealing with lesbian or gay people should examine the reasons and find ways to ensure that homosexual patients are not disadvantaged.

Sexuality has been a neglected area of nurse education, and many nurses do not feel comfortable discussing issues relating to sex. Every nurse needs to have come to terms with her/his own feelings before being able to help the patients. The degree of involvement in sexual health issues will vary with the knowledge and expertise of individual nurses.

Relationships

Nurses should be aware of the many ways in which patients can experience problems:

- *Ignorance* – about the way the body functions, or how the emotions can affect sexual functioning.
- *Lack of self-esteem* – not being able to say 'no', or to refuse unsafe sex.
- *Effects of illness, drugs, or disability* – carers can experience a role conflict when expected to be both nurse and lover. Medication such as beta-blockers can cause impotence. Patients recovering from a heart attack may fear a recurrence with any exertion. Patients with severe arthritis, paraplegia or other disabilities, may have practical problems with sexual performance.
- *Loneliness* – in patients without a partner, can lead to depression and a lack of purpose in life[3].

Patients with some of these problems may need specialised help, but a practice nurse who recognises that need can offer appropriate information or counselling, or refer elsewhere as appropriate.

Education for nurses

The family planning courses approved by the National Boards (ENB901 in England) provide a broad education in issues concerned with sexual health, fertility and contraception. Other specialised courses can be undertaken in sexually transmitted diseases, fertility care and psycho-sexual counselling.

Family planning nurses are required to keep their knowledge and skills up-to-date[4]. The RCN Family Planning Nurses Forum runs study days, issues a newsletter for members and has produced the booklet *Standards of Care for Family Planning Nurses*. The RCN *Family Planning Manual for Nurses* describes practical procedures in detail. The Family Planning Association produces a wide range of useful literature and a quarterly bulletin, *Family Planning Today*.

Family planning

Family planning should not be considered to be an exclusively female concern. Couples may attend the surgery together to discuss contraception, preparation for pregnancy, infertility, or sterilisation.

Some patients prefer to visit a DHA Family Planning Clinic because it offers anonymity. Adolescents may fear that the GP will tell their parents about the consultation[5]. Practice nurses can offer reassurance that the service is strictly confidential and will not be discussed with anyone without the consent of the patient. The law on the provision of contraceptive advice to children under 16 was clarified as a result of the Gillick Case[6]. Parental responsibility should not be undermined and whenever possible the young person should be persuaded to tell a parent or guardian, but if for example family relationships have broken down, a doctor or nurse would not be acting unlawfully if the young person:

- was sufficiently mature to understand all the implications,
- would not allow a parent to know that contraceptive advice was being sought,
- would be very likely to have sexual intercourse without contraception.

When a doctor or nurse first sees any patient for contraceptive advice a number of aspects need to be considered.

General assessment of the patient

- *general medical history* – to identify any contraindications to specific methods of contraception,
- *obstetric and gynaecological history* – including menses, pregnancies, rubella status, cervical screening,
- *personal history* – because smoking, lifestyle or relationships may influence the choice of method,
- *family history* – in case the patient may have an inherited susceptibility to CVS disease, diabetes or cancer,
- *measurement of BP, weight and height* – as part of the general health

assessment. Also because hormone contraception can cause weight gain and elevation of the blood pressure,

- *cervical screening, pelvic and breast examination* – as appropriate.

The criteria for contraception

There is no perfect method of contraception. The points to consider when choosing a method include:

- *safety* of the method and any potential health risks,
- *efficacy and reliability* of the method,
- *acceptability* to both partners,
- *availability* – where and how easily it can be obtained,
- *cost* – if any.

Counselling

Patients should be able to make their own decisions after receiving adequate information and the chance to explore any fears or anxieties. It is important not to impose one's own values and judgements. *Your Guide to Contraception*, a leaflet produced by the Family Planning Association explains all the methods currently available – how they work, their reliability, advantages and disadvantages and other relevant information. The leaflet can be used as a basis for discussion when helping patients to compare the different methods.

The methods available

Oral contraception

There are many formulations of 'the pill' but they can be grouped into two distinct types:

- the combined oral contraceptive pill,
- the progestogen only pill.

The doctor will prescribe the appropriate type of pill after a discussion with the patient and consideration of any contraindications.

The combined oral contraceptive pill (COC)

COCs contain oestrogen and progestogen and act by inhibiting ovulation. A pill is taken daily for 21 days followed by 7 pill-free days. A withdrawal bleed usually occurs during this week. If any pills are missed – especially at the beginning or end of a packet to lengthen the number of pill-free days, then ovulation and pregnancy can occur.

The combined pill is often the first choice of younger women, for whom convenience and reliability rate highly. COCs can increase the risk of thrombo-embolism, so may be contraindicated for some patients.

Phasic pills contain varying hormone strengths which are intended to mimic the natural cycle. Phasic pills have been thought to give a better bleeding pattern, but more pill-taking errors can occur[7].

Every day (ED) pills contain seven placebo pills to be taken after the 21 active pills. They are useful for patients who forget to restart a packet after a week's break, but the pills must be taken in the correct order.

Emergency hormone contraception can be prescribed up to 72 hours after unprotected intercourse. Ethinyloestrodiol 50mcg and levo-norgestrol 250mcg (e.g. PC4 or Ovran) two to be taken immediately and repeated after 12 hours. The pills can cause nausea and if vomiting occurs a dose may need to be repeated. Mifepristone (RU468) in a single dose has been shown to produce less side-effects and be more effective in preventing pregnancy[8]. Suitable methods of contraception need to be discussed, and the patient must attend for follow up after three weeks. A pregnancy test should be performed if the period does not start when expected.

The progestogen only pill (POP)

POPs act by making the cervical mucus inpenetrable to sperm, and by changing the endometrium to prevent a fertilised ovum being implanted. The pills must be taken at the same time (or within three hours) every day, without a break, in order to maintain these physiological effects.

The bleeding pattern may be more erratic than with the COC pill, and weight gain or mood changes may make the method less well-tolerated. POPs do not carry a thrombotic risk, so are more suitable for older women, heavy smokers and others who cannot be prescribed the combined pill. POPs can also be taken by breast-feeding mothers.

Oral contraceptive routines

Each practice should have agreed guidelines for dealing both with patients who need oral contraception for the first time, and for those who need follow-up appointments.

First-time pill users

New pill users require education about:

- how the pill works and affects the body,
- how to take the pill and when to start (day 1 of cycle will give immediate contraceptive protection),
- what to do if a pill is missed (see Fig. 12.1),

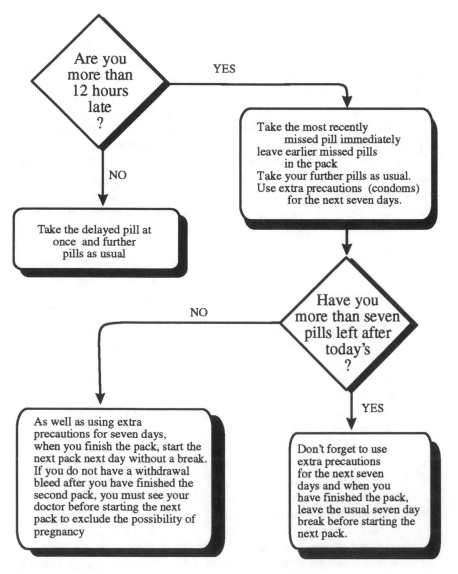

Fig. 12.1   Missed pill guidelines.

- how diarrhoea and vomiting or some medicines and antibiotics can prevent the pill from being absorbed; so extra precautions need to be taken,
- how to recognise any abnormal effects and when to contact the GP,
- the risk of sexually transmitted diseases and the use of condoms for protection.

There is too much information for a patient to remember after being told once, so appropriate instruction sheets should also be provided. The doctor or nurse must check that the patient understands the information given.

Patients already taking the pill

New pill users should return after three months, when BP, weight and bleeding should be recorded, and any problems or worries discussed. Established pill users require a 'pill-check' at least once a year. Regular cervical smears should be taken once a woman has been sexually active for about a year[9].

The patient's knowledge and understanding of her pill use should be checked to ensure that no essential information has been forgotten or misunderstood.

Barrier methods

The diaphragm and cap

In general practice the diaphragm (often called 'the cap') is a commonly prescribed barrier method. Diaphragms are made of thin latex rubber, in a range of sizes. Each one has a flexible wire inside the rim to make it fit comfortably into the vagina. The cervical cap, vault cap or vimule may be used by women whose anatomy makes diaphragm use difficult (see Fig. 12.2). They all need to be used with a spermicide. The patient needs to be taught how to use the diaphragm, by a family planning-trained doctor or nurse. The teaching should cover:

- how to locate the cervix,
- how and when to insert the diaphragm or cap and to check that the cervix is covered (Fig. 12.3),
- to use extra spermicide if more than three hours since the 'cap' was inserted, or intercourse last occurred,
- how and when to remove the device (six hours must elapse after intercourse),

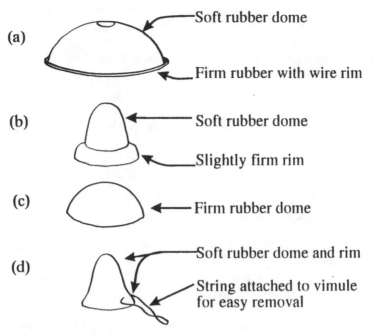

(a) Diaphragm dutch cap.   (b) Cervical cap.   (c) Vault or Dumas cap.   (d) Vimule cap.

Fig. 12.2   Types of cap.

- how to look after the 'cap' and check for any damage or perishing,
- when to return for a check or re-fitting (annual checks or if a significant weight change or pregnancy occurs),
- how to obtain emergency contraception if needed.

The diaphragm is a popular method with many women for whom the pill is unacceptable or contraindicated. The method may not be suitable for a woman who is unhappy about feeling for her cervix, who has very lax pelvic floor muscles, or who suffers from recurrent symptoms of cystitis or thrush. Some patients may be allergic to the spermicide.

Male and female condoms

Male condoms have had significant publicity since the advent of HIV and AIDS. Free condoms are issued at family planning and GUM clinics but unfortunately, few GPs are able to provide them too. Patients need to be reminded about the protection condoms can offer against sexually

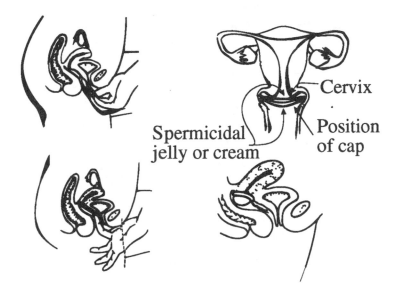

Spermicidal jelly or cream

Cervix

Position of cap

Fig. 12.3 Insertion and correct position of the cap.

transmitted diseases and of the correct way to apply a condom. The following points are essential:

- Make sure the condom has been stored properly and is not past its 'sell by date'.
- Open the foil wrap carefully so the condom is not damaged.
- Expel the air from the teat at the end of the condom, to allow room for the ejaculate.
- Roll the condom onto the erect penis before any contact with the female genital area takes place.
- Hold the condom in place and withdraw the penis before it becomes flaccid after ejaculation.
- Dispose of used condoms safely. Wrap it in a tissue and place in a bin. Do not flush it down the toilet.
- Make sure a female partner knows about emergency contraception if a condom fails.

The female condom is a fairly recent innovation which has not yet achieved widespread popularity. The condom is a soft latex sac with a polythene ring inside to help the insertion of the condom into the vagina, and a fixed ring around the opening which lies over the labia. It provides

additional protection against genital herpes and other sexually transmitted diseases. These condoms can be bought in pharmacies.

The sponge

The sponge is a small device impregnated with spermicide which is
placed in the vagina across the cervix. The sponge can be bought in
pharmacies, is easy to use and does not require special instruction. It
should be moistened with water before being inserted. The method has a
high failure rate and is only recommended for use by women who would
not really mind becoming pregnant, or possibly for women approaching
the menopause, when fertility is lessened.

The intrauterine device (IUD)

The method, also known as 'the coil', involves the insertion of a small
plastic and copper device into the uterus where it acts by preventing the
establishment of a fertilised ovum in the endometrium. New progestogen
releasing IUDs are undergoing trials in the United Kingdom. Fine nylon
threads, attached to the end of the IUD, pass through the cervix to aid
the removal of the device. The commonly used copper-bearing devices
are shown in Fig. 12.4 . The IUD is more suitable for multiparous women
because the slightly increased risk of pelvic infection could threaten the
future fertility of women without children. The device must be inserted
by a doctor, but the nurse will usually prepare the equipment, assist as
needed, and look after the patient throughout the procedure (see
Chapter 5). Patients can imagine tremendous horrors, so it is worth
keeping some unsterile IUDS to demonstrate to patients what the coil
looks like, where it is put, and how it works.

There may be slight cramp-like pain immediately after the insertion, as
the uterus tries to expel the IUD. A mild analgesic may be given. The
patient should be allowed to rest for a while, and during this time the
nurse can teach her how to feel the threads coming out from the cervix.
If the patient can feel the threads each month after menstruation she will
know the device is still in place and has not been expelled during the
menstrual period.

The patient needs to have clear information about the possible
immediate and long-term effects, and when to consult the doctor. The
slight abdominal discomfort usually settles within a day or so. Periods
may be heavier for a while, and the device could be expelled. Consult the
doctor if low abdominal pain or vaginal discharge occur – there may be
some pelvic infection.

Emergency contraception can be providedd by an IUD inserted up to

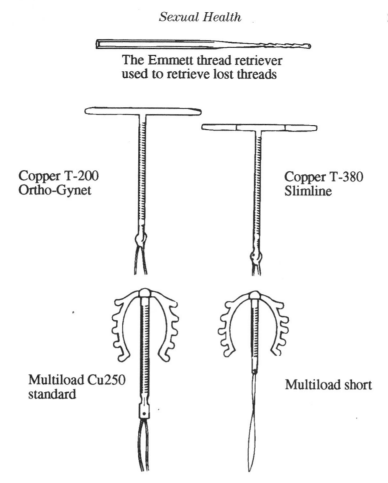

The Emmett thread retriever
used to retrieve lost threads

Copper T-200
Ortho-Gynet

Copper T-380
Slimline

Multiload Cu250
standard

Multiload short

Fig. 12.4 IUCDs commonly used in general practice.

five days after unprotected intercourse, to prevent the implantation of a
fertilised ovum. The IUD may be removed if necessary once the risk of
pregnancy is past, but suitable alternative contraception should also be
arranged.

Injectable methods

The most commonly used injectable progestogen is Depo-Provera
150mg given by deep intramuscular injection every 12 weeks. This is
normally given in the first five days of the cycle. It can also be injected
within five days of a miscarriage or abortion, or five weeks after childbirth. The method is useful for women with erratic lifestyles who forget
to take the pill and cannot cope with other methods. It is worthwhile to

keep a record of patients receiving contraceptive injections as some may need reminding when the next injection is due.

The disadvantages include:

- Once injected the hormone cannot be removed, so any side-effects must be tolerated for up to 12 weeks.
- Patients can suffer weight gain, mood changes or erratic bleeding.
- With repeated injections patients tend to become amenorrhoeic, often with a delayed return to fertility.

Implants

Many GPs are learning how to insert long-acting hormone implants. Norplant became available in the UK in October 1993. Six silastic rods which contain levonorgestrol are implanted in a fan shape under the skin of the upper, inner arm. The progestogen is released slowly over five years and acts by inhibiting ovulation and by making the cervical mucus inpenetrable to sperm. The rods can be removed at any time so that their effect can be reversed. The patients need careful counselling about the method, and possible effects on the bleeding pattern.

Natural methods

Religious or personal reasons may lead some couples to opt for natural family planning. A high level of motivation is required and special teaching is essential. Couples can avoid intercourse once they have learned to identify the fertile time each month (Fig. 12.5). Various methods may be used – often in combination:

- *Calendar.* Keeping records of the menstrual cycle. Ovulation occurs approximately 14 days before the menstrual period starts.
- *Temperature.* This method uses very careful recordings of the body temperature each day, using a special fertility thermometer, to identify the slight temperature rise which occurs at ovulation. (Febrile illness will nullify the readings.)
- *Cervical mucus.* This can be used to recognise the fertile time because the consistency and amount of the mucus changes around the time of ovulation (to facilitate the entry of spermatazoa).
- Commercially available test kits. These detect ovulation by the surge in luteinising hormone, but do not yet predict ovulation early enough to be reliable for contraception.

The success or failure of natural methods relies on being able to predict

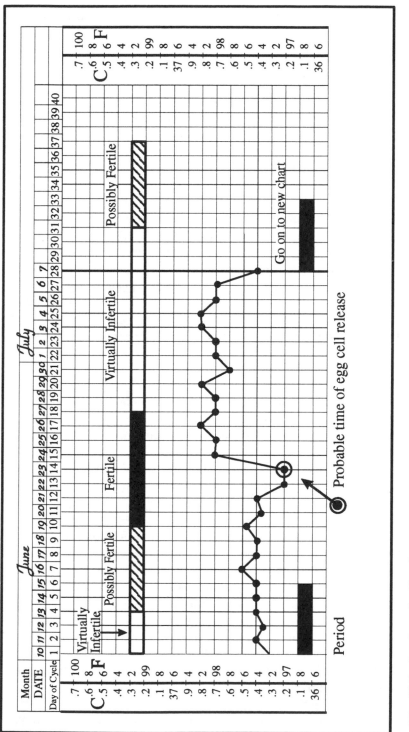

Fig. 12.5 Specimen fertility chart.

ovulation accurately so that intercourse is avoided for at least five days before and three days afterwards.

Male and female sterilisation

Sterilisation is the ultimate contraception. It should be regarded as permanent even though advances in microsurgery might make reversal possible. Couples who have completed their families may opt for this method, but with divorce and second marriages now so common, they need to consider all the possible eventualities before reaching a decision about sterilisation.

Vasectomy

Sterilisation for the male entails cutting the spermatic cord just as it enters the inguinal canal after leaving the scrotum. It is an easy operation which can be performed under local anaesthetic as an out-patient. Some GPs will perform vasectomies in the surgery. The patient should be advised not to undertake strenuous physical activity for a few days, to reduce the possibility of bruising around the operation site. The following points should be emphasised when discussing this method of sterilisation with patients:

- It is permanent, but not until two consecutive sperm counts are negative.
- There will be no adverse effect on erection, sexual performance, or ejaculation.
- As the majority of the ejaculate is made up of secretions from the prostate and other glands the patient will notice little change after the operation.

Semen samples are required monthly for three to four months after the operation. Contraceptive precautions must be continued until two consecutive samples contain no sperm. There has been some concern about an increased risk of prostatic cancer after vasectomy but no evidence has been found to support this[10].

Female sterilisation

A woman is sterilised by cutting or clipping the fallopian tubes so that the ovum cannot pass down them into the uterus. The vast majority of female sterilisations are carried out under general anaesthetic using a laparoscope. Patients should be warned to expect some discomfort until the gas introduced into the peritoneal cavity to make the pelvic organs accessible, has dispersed. The practice nurse may be required to remove the sutures from the small abdominal incision sites.

Education

Any method of contraception may fail if the user does not learn everything he or she needs to know about using the method safely. Doctors and nurses who provide family planning services need to have enough time, appropriate visual aids, and be able to choose suitable teaching styles for each patient.

Administrative aspects

Patients who receive contraceptive advice or treatment by a GP or family planning nurse must also have regular reviews. This means that the patient's record must show what method is being used and when the next check is due. The GP can claim item of service fees for providing family planning services, so the relevant forms must be completed and despatched to ensure that practice income is not lost:

- *FP1001* – is signed annually by all patients who have been offered contraception or advice about contraceptive methods.
- *FP1002* – a fee claim for the insertion of an IUD. Thereafter an annual fee is claimed on FP1001 for the annual IUD check. An FP1002 can only be claimed once in a year, even if an IUD is fitted more than once in that year.
- *FP1003* – a fee claim for giving contraceptive advice to a temporary patient.

Patients are allowed to consult any GP for contraceptive advice without having to be registered at that practice. This can be useful when a patient is embarrassed about seeing a GP who is an old family friend. It is important for reception staff to be aware of this ruling, so that they do not turn patients away.

Termination of pregnancy

It is vital that nobody enters a sexual relationship with the attitude that 'if anything goes wrong an abortion can be arranged'. Apart from the undesirability of using termination as a form of contraception, there are health risks which include:

- a higher incidence of pelvic inflammatory disease,
- cervical incompetence in future wanted pregnancies,
- the usual operative risks of anaesthesia and of haemorrhage,
- the psychological consequences.

The decision of a doctor to refer a woman for a termination will depend on a number of factors which can only be taken into account after careful discussion and counselling. The law requires that a statement be completed by two doctors (preferably the GP and the gynaecologist) who have to state that the patient falls into one of four categories:

- The continuation of the pregnancy would involve risk to the life of the pregnant woman greater than if the pregnancy was terminated.
- The continuance of the pregnancy would involve risk of injury to the physical or mental health of the pregnant woman greater than if the pregnancy was terminated.
- The continuance of the pregnancy would involve risk of injury to the physical or mental health of the pregnant woman or any existing child(ren) of her family greater than if the pregnancy was terminated.
- There is substantial risk that if the child was born it would suffer from such physical and mental abnormalities as to be severely handicapped[11].

The termination itself may be performed within the NHS or privately. (Abortion is not available in Northern Ireland – except in very exceptional circumstances.) All patients who have a termination must be encouraged to undertake ways of preventing further unwanted pregnancies. The decision to have an abortion can be traumatic and cause mental distress at any time after the event. A practice nurse might be able to give support or counselling and should know where to refer a patient if help is needed.

The moral and ethical aspects of termination have not been considered here because each reader will have his or her own opinion on this emotive subject. However, the UKCC requires nurses to promote and safeguard the interest and well-being of their patients and clients, and to ensure that no act or omission within the nurse's sphere of responsibility is detrimental to a patient's interest, condition or safety[12].

Sexually transmitted diseases

The risks of acquiring a sexually transmitted disease (STD) should be explained when discussing contraception or sexual health issues. Chlamydia, genital warts, herpes, HIV and hepatitis B can all be transmitted sexually; not just syphilis and gonorrhoea.

A patient with symptoms of a sexually transmitted disease should be advised to attend the Genito-Urinary Medicine (GUM) Clinic; where the facilities exist for prompt diagnosis and treatment as well as counselling and contact-tracing. Practice nurses can help by providing information about the clinic times and location, and reassuring patients about the confidentiality maintained there.

More patients with human immunodeficiency (HIV) infection are being seen in general practice these days, but sadly some practices will still not allow them to register. Such patients pose no health risk, providing the guidelines outlined in Chapter 4 are followed.

The majority of people with HIV infection are asymptomatic. The progression of the disease to Acquired Immune Deficiency Syndrome (AIDS) varies from person to person. Persistent generalised lymphadenopathy, or generalised symptoms related to immune deficiency – severe diarrhoea and weight loss, fatigue, night sweats, candidiasis, and herpes may first point to a diagnosis of HIV infection.

Opportunistic diseases which would normally be overcome by the T4 cells can become life-threatening. Pneumocystis carinii pneumonia (PCP), cytomegalovirus infection, tuberculosis, and Karposi's sarcoma are diagnostic of AIDS in HIV positive patients. Neurological involvement can lead to loss of motor or sensory function and dementia.

Better drugs and technology are allowing many patients to live for longer periods with HIV infection, but they also require extra support and kindness. Voluntary organisations exist for HIV positive men, women, children, partners, and members of ethnic groups and religions. Practice nurses can assist by treating patients with HIV as any other patients who need help or advice, and by educating other people about the disease. The local HIV/AIDS adviser will provide any extra training needed.

Suggestions for evaluation and research

- Review your professional profile:
    (a) What training/education have you received on human sexuality? Was it adequate for dealing with patients on the subject without feeling embarassed? What further training do you think you need?
    (b) Were you taught to consider that patients might not be

heterosexual when you are talking with them? Reflect on ways of treating all people equally.

- Audit the patients fitted with a diaphragm or cap. How many return for 'cap' checks when they are due?
- Compile a questionnaire to find out how many patients taking the oral contraceptive know what to do if they miss a pill or have a gastric upset. How could patient education be improved?
- Conduct a search of recent literature on HIV/AIDS. How might the knowledge affect your nursing practice?

References

1. Masters, W. and Johnson, W. (1966) *Human Sexual Response*. Little Brown and Co., Boston.
2. Savage, J. (1987) *Nurses, Gender and Sexuality*. Heinemann Medical Books, London.
3. Callaghan, P. and Morrissey, M. (1993) Social support and health: a review; *Journal of Advanced Nursing* **18:** 203–210.
4. Royal College of Nursing (1989) *Standards of Care: Family Planning Nursing;* Professional and ethical matters: 4. Scutari Press, Harrow.
5. Francome, C. (1994) Why teenagers do not trust GPs; *GP*, January 14: 46.
6. DHSS (1986) Family Planning Services for young people; Health Circular HC(86)1. DHSS, London.
7. Guillebaud, J. (1993) *Contraception – Your Questions Answered* (2nd Edn): 189–190. Churchill Livingstone, Edinburgh.
8. Webb, A.M.C., Russell, J. and Elstein, M. (1992) Comparison of Yupze regimen, danazol and mefipristone (RU486) in oral post-coital contraception; *British Medical Journal*, **305:** 927–931.
9. Kleinman, R. (Ed.) (1980) *Family Planning Handbook for Doctors*: 198. IPPF.
10. Nienhuis, H., Goldacre, M., Seagroatt, V., Leicester, G. and Versey, M. (1992) Incidence of disease after vasectomy – a record linkage retrospective cohort study; *British Medical Journal* **304:** 743–746.
11. Great Britain, Parliament (1990) *The Abortion Act 1967, amended by the Human Fertilisation and Embryology Act 1990*. HMSO, London.
12. UKCC (1992) *Code of Professional Conduct* (3rd Edn): 1.2.UKCC, London.

Further reading

Gamel, C., Davis, B.D. and Hengeveld, M. (1993) Nurses' provision of teaching and counselling on sexuality: a review of the literature; *Journal of Advanced Nursing*, **18:** 1219–1227.

Webb, C. (1985) *Sexuality, Nursing and Health*. John Wiley & Sons, Chichester.

Norris, S. and Read, E. (1985) *Out in the Open – People Talking about Being Gay or Bisexual.* Pan Books, London.

Family Planning Association (1993) *FPA Factfile: a Series of Factsheets on Contraception, Sexuality and Sex Education.* FPA, London.

Useful addresses

Association to Aid the Sexual and Personal Relationships of the Disabled (SPOD)
286 Camden Road, London N7 0BJ.

Family Planning Association
27–35 Mortimer Street, London W1N 7RJ.
Telephone 071-636 7866. *Fax* 071-436 3288.

National AIDS Helpline
PO Box 1577, London NW1 3DW.
Telephone 0800-567123.

Chapter 13
Women's Health

Nearly all practice nurses are female[1]. This can give an advantage when dealing with women's health issues because many patients feel more comfortable talking to another woman[2]. The expectation by society that women should care for others – partners, children, elderly parents, can mean they have little time left to care for themselves. A practice nurse who shows a friendly concern can allow women to put their own interests first for a while.

Well-woman screening involves factors related to the female reproductive function in addition to the general health screening outlined in Chapter 9. A thorough history should be obtained to ensure that every patient receives the appropriate care and advice.

Menstruation

Nurses need to be aware of the range of normal menstrual cycles for different women in order to recognise any abnormalities of menstruation. There may be considerable variations in cycle length and menstrual flow but an average normal pattern can be considered as:

- *The start of menstrual periods (menarche)* age 10–13 years. They may be irregular at first but settle into a regular cycle by about 16 years.
- *A menstrual cycle* of approximately 28 days with bleeding over 4–5 days. (The first day of bleeding is calculated as day 1 of the cycle).
- *The cessation of menstrual periods (menopause)* at about 48–52 years.

A nurse can help a woman with concerns about menstruation by:

- getting the patient to give a clear outline of the problem,
- checking on the patient's knowledge and understanding of menstruation,

- showing her how to keep a menstrual chart and encouraging her to consult the GP with it, if necessary,
- giving practical advice for dealing with discomfort, and using appropriate sanitary protection.

Young women should be taught why menstruation is a normal event rather than a 'curse', but women who do have problems with menstruation deserve sympathetic understanding.

Dysmenorrhoea

Painful periods cause misery for some women each month. Exercise can often relieve the cramp-like pain of normal periods, and mild analgesics may help. Mefanamic acid (Ponstan) may be prescribed for more severe pain. Secondary dysmenorrhoea requiring medical investigation can be caused by an IUD, pelvic inflammatory disease, endometriosis or fibroids.

Menorrhagia

Heavy bleeding can be distressing and embarrassing. Abnormal pathology needs to be ruled out and the extent of the problem needs to be assessed. Patients can be asked to record the number of pads or tampons used, the frequency of change and any clots passed. Heavy irregular bleeding may develop in the perimenopausal years. A haemoglobin estimation should be made if anaemia is suspected.

Amenorrhoea

Pregnancy is a common cause of absent periods. Other causes include: anxiety, moving to a new environment, examination stress, excessive dieting and exercise, anaemia, and endocrine diseases. Secondary amenorrhoea can result from hormone contraceptive use.

Pre-menstrual syndrome (PMS)

Most women experience some physiological changes during the latter half of the menstrual cycle. Breast tenderness, fluid retention or mood changes are a response to the changing hormone levels. More extreme symptoms are termed pre-menstrual syndrome. PMS has even been used as a legal defence by women accused of crimes like shop-lifting or motoring offences[3]. Practice nurses can help patients to talk about their problems and encourage them to keep a diary of their symptoms in relation to the menstrual cycle.

The symptoms may be helped by diet and exercise. Coffee should be restricted because the caffeine may increase irritability. A low salt intake may reduce fluid retention, and diuretics can be prescribed by the GP if necessary. Pyridoxine (vitamin B6), oil of evening primrose, the contraceptive pill, or progesterone suppositories may help some patients.

Cervical cytology

Cervical smears are taken to detect any pre-malignant changes in the cells of the cervix; cervical intra-epithelial neoplasia (CIN), which might develop into invasive cancer if not treated. The cytology report will indicate the severity of any changes and suggest when the test should be repeated, or if the patient should be referred for colposcopy. The reduction of death from cervical cancer is one of the targets in *The Health of the Nation*.

Targets

GPs are paid for meeting a target of 70%, or a lower target of 50% for cervical screening for women aged 20 to 65 years. A good administration system is needed to maintain the practice income, but the prime concern should be for the welfare of women. Younger women are not included in the smear targets but regular smears are advisable once a girl has been sexually active for about a year. As with many screening activities, those most at risk are often the least likely to attend[4]. Opportunistic screening is needed in addition to an effective call and recall system.

Practice nurses can help to reduce the anxiety associated with cervical screening, but any nurse involved must have had the necessary theoretical and practical experience and be accountable for her practice. The degree of nurse involvement will depend on the level of knowledge and expertise. The RCN has issued guidelines for good practice in cervical screening[5].

- *Level 1*. Administration – checking when smears are due and reminding patients when they are seen for other purposes. Educating patients about cervical screening and providing appropriate literature for them to read.
- *Level 2*. As in *Level 1* plus:
  Taking an appropriate history and completing the smear form with all the relevant personal details, and comprehensive information about previous smears. Taking a satisfactory cervical smear (see Chapter

5). Making sure the patient knows how to get the result of the test and that a contact address is known. Interpreting an abnormal smear result to a patient.

- *Level 3.* As in *Levels 1 and 2* plus:
  Performing a bi-manual pelvic examination to detect any tenderness or masses in the pelvic organs, if appropriate.

Laboratories vary in the terminology used to describe cervical cell changes. Nurses should ask for clarification from their local department of cytology. Smears may be described as:

- *Inadequate* – due to insufficient cells on the slide, cells obscured by blood or mucus, or poor fixation.
- *Negative* – no abnormality detected.
- *No endocervical cells seen* – the sample may not have contained cells from the squamo-columnar junction (the transformation zone), where pre-malignant changes most commonly occur.
- *Inflammatory* – cell changes due to infection or irritation of the cervix.
- *Borderline dyskaryosis* – some atypical cells seen.
- *Mild dyskariosis or CIN 1* – changes in the nucleus of some cells.
- *Moderate dyskariosis or CIN 2* – more marked changes in the nuclei.
- *Severe dyskaryosis or CIN 3* – a larger number of cells with grossly abnormal nuclei.
- *Malignant cells present* – suggestive of invasive cancer[6].

Patients with borderline or mild changes will be recalled for repeat smears after 3–12 months. After several borderline results or if CIN 2 or 3 is found the patient will be referred to a gynaecologist for colposcopy. A booklet *The Abnormal Smear*, explains to patients the procedure of colposcopy and the treatment of abnormal cells[7]. Colposcopy means looking directly at the cervix with a special microscope attached to a vaginal speculum. The cervix is stained with iodine or acetic acid to delineate any areas of abnomality and a biopsy can be taken. Abnormal cells can be destroyed by laser cautery or cryosurgery. Occasionally a cone biopsy may be performed under general anaesthetic to remove abnormal cells which extend into the cervical canal. Patients who have had treatment for CIN must have regular smear tests and follow-up.

Breast examination

Breast cancer is the largest single cause of death of women in the UK. One target of the government's health strategy is a 25% reduction in such deaths by the year 2000. Patients with several close female relatives who have had the disease may be referred to a breast unit for regular screening. All women need to understand the importance of recognising any change in their breasts and of seeking medical help quickly.

Practice nurses can teach '*breast awareness*' to their patients. The principles include:

- *Looking at the breasts.* This is to detect anything unusual (change in the outline, dimpling of the skin, retraction or change in a nipple). A patient should do this in front of a mirror with her arms at the sides, then raised above the head, and finally with her hands pressed onto the hips to accentuate the breast contours.
- *Feeling the breast tissue.* The patient should lie flat with her head on a pillow and a towel or small pillow under the shoulder of the side to be examined. Using the flat of the fingers together and working systematically around all the breast tissue and into the axilla, the breast tissue should be compressed firmly but gently against the chest wall. The nipple should be sqeezed gently to see if any blood or discharge is expressed.

A doctor should be consulted immediately if any abnormality is supected.

The National Health Service breast screening service

Women aged 50–64 are offered mammography every three years. The screening programme has only been in operation since 1990 but a significant number of early cancers are being picked up[8]. Nurses can encourage their patients to attend, and reassure them that the procedure only takes a few moments. It entails stripping to the waist and standing next to an X-ray machine while the breast is compressed between two special plates. This can be rather uncomfortable but only lasts for a few seconds while the X-ray is taken. If further tests are needed the patient will be invited to see the specialist at her local breast unit. Explanatory leaflets are available from regional breast screening centres.

Women over 64 are not invited but will be screened if they request it. Women under 50 are not yet eligible for the programme, although screening may be offered to younger women in the future. Women of any age who have symptoms should consult their GP because the national screening programme is only intended for asymptomatic women. Although breast screening may ultimately save lives, the unexpected diagnosis of cancer can be devastating. Such patients require skilled counselling and support.

Pre-conceptual care

Patients may ask for advice about the best ways to prepare for pregnancy. Such advice for both partners should cover lifestyle factors and the avoidance of known hazards. Healthy living means not smoking tobacco, severely restricting alcohol intake, having regular exercise and adequate sleep, and eating a well-balanced diet (see Chapter 9). Folic acid is particularly important because a deficiency is thought to contribute to neural tube defects[9]. Foods rich in folic acid include: dark leafy vegetables, oranges, beans, fortified bread and breakfast cereals, beef and yeast extracts.

Blood should be taken to test for rubella antibodies if a woman's immunity has not been confirmed. If a patient needs to be immunised against rubella she must be warned to avoid becoming pregnant for at least one month after immunisation[10]. Any occupational hazards to pregnant women should be identified, and a transfer may have to be considered at work. Radiation and anaesthetic gases, for example, are known to be hazardous[11].

Any medicines a patient takes should be checked to ensure they will not harm the foetus. Some changes to medication may be necessary. Patients who are planning to travel abroad should be made aware of any health risks. Careful planning of immunisations and anti-malarial prophylaxis is needed. Mefloquine is contraindicated if pregnancy could possibly occur within three months of taking the tablets.

It may be necessary to check the patient's understanding of the menstrual cycle and when ovulation is most likely to occur. The natural methods of contraception (see Chapter 12) can also help patients who *want* to conceive to recognise their fertile time.

Patients with any family or personal history of a hereditary condition may be referred to a specialist for genetic counselling.

Infertility

Patients who are unable to have children may consult their GP for help. Most couples will be referred to a fertility specialist, but the practice nurse may be involved with some of the fertility tests or with giving pre-conceptual health advice. The RCN Fertility Nurses Group booklet *Standards of Care for Fertility Nurses* can also be helpful for practice nurses.

Patients who embark on the stressful process of investigation and treatment of infertility will require patience and commitment. A sense of humour also helps. Specialist infertility centres must employ counsellors[12], but practice nurses can also help by listening to patients' concerns, being sympathetic to their needs, and making sure they have received all the information they require.

Male patients may visit the practice nurse for testosterone injections to improve the quality of spermatazoa. Female patients may require injections of gonadotrophin to stimulate ovulation. They can be rather painful, so a sympathetic approach is needed.

In vitro fertilisation (IVF) and embryo transfer.

Drugs are used to stimulate several ova to ripen at once. This is carefully monitored by blood tests and ultrasound and at the appropriate time the mature eggs are collected via a laparoscope and placed in a culture medium. Specially prepared sperm collected from the partner's semen are added to the ova in the containers. Once fertilisation has occurred, the selected embryos are introduced through the cervix into the patient's uterus. Progesterone injections or pessaries may be given to assist the implantation. Extra embryos may be deep frozen for future use in case the pregnancy does not become established.

Gamete intra-fallopian transfer (GIFT)

This is a procedure similar to IVF except that the ova and sperm are mixed and transferred to the fallopian tube before fertilisation.

Pregnancy

A practice nurse may be the first person to confirm a pregnancy after performing the pregnancy test. First time parents will welcome some information about what to expect. The pregnancy is counted from the first day of the last menstrual period, so the expected date of delivery can be calculated as 40 weeks from then. Special calculator discs are available for this purpose. A copy of the most recent edition of *The New Pregnancy Book*[13] can be supplied. It gives very clear information about all the aspects of pregnancy. A booklet on maternity benefits can also be provided[14]. Smoking and a high alcohol intake in pregnancy are known to be harmful[15,16]. The opportunity should be taken to advise on their avoidance or restriction. Soft cheeses, pâté and under-cooked meat should be avoided because of the risk of listeria infection[17]. A high intake of vitamin A can also be dangerous, so pregnant women should be advised not to eat liver or large quantities of vitamin A supplements[18].

Maternity care

The arrangements for maternity care can differ from area to area, so it is worthwhile for a practice nurse to familiarise herself with the arrangements locally. Shared care between the GP, the community midwife and the obstetrician is often popular. Some GPs provide medical cover for home confinements.

Antenatal care

Practice nurses may assist with some aspects of antenatal care. A patient will attend the first antenatal clinic when she is approximately 12 weeks pregnant. The midwife obtains a full medical and obstetric history, which is summarised on a co-operation obstetric record card. The patient carries the card with her to all hospital and clinic appointments throughout the pregnancy. The height, weight and blood pressure are recorded, and the urine is tested for glucose and albumin. Blood tests are taken for full blood count (FBC), blood group, rubella antibodies and syphilis. The GP may perform a medical examination. The appropriate booking is made for home, GP unit or hospital confinement, and the patient is given a certificate of eligibility for free dental care and prescriptions.

The patient returns for further antenatal checks at monthly intervals until about 30 weeks pregnant, then fortnightly until 36 weeks, and weekly thereafter. There may be local variations in the investigations performed, but the following is a guide:

- 16–18 weeks – blood tests for neural tube defect (AFP) and Downs screening.
- 18 weeks – routine ultrasound scan.
- 28 weeks – FBC, blood group and antibodies.
- 34 weeks – FBC, blood group and antibodies.

After 24 weeks pregnancy a certificate (MatB1) is issued, which entitles a woman to maternity benefits.

Postnatal care

The patient attends for a full postnatal examination about six weeks after confinement. The haemoglobin may be checked, and rubella immunisation given, if needed. A routine cervical smear is usually taken at this time. The doctor should complete the maternity claim form (FP24).

Contraception should be discussed and appropriate arrangements made. Oral contraception can be started right away, but the progestogen-only pill must be used while the patient is breast-feeding. An IUD or diaphragm can be fitted if preferred.

Lax pelvic floor muscles contribute to urinary incontinence and uterine prolapse. The patient should be encouraged to continue post-natal exercises to regain muscle tone:

- Lie on the couch, lift both legs straight up; slowly lower them to the couch; repeat ten times twice daily.
- Once a day stop midstream for a short while during micturition, then complete the stream.
- Tighten the buttock and perineal muscles when standing. (This can be performed as many times as possible during the day, even when performing household chores.)

Practice nurses usually have a peripheral role in pre- and postnatal care, but such contacts offer the chance to establish a good relationship so the parent will be less anxious about bringing the baby for immunisation.

Miscarriage

There can be many mishaps between conception and the delivery of a healthy infant. An anxious patient may telephone the practice nurse for advice if the doctor is unavailable.

Bleeding in the early months of pregnancy may settle down, but patients need support while they wait to see what happens. Although rest probably won't affect the outcome, it can help women to feel they did everything possible if the pregnancy is lost. The doctor will usually arrange an urgent ultrasound scan, but admission to hospital will be needed if the bleeding is severe. A woman with a rhesus negative blood group must be given an injection of anti-D immunoglobulin within 72 hours of a miscarriage; to prevent the development of antibodies which could affect a subsequent foetus.

The Stillbirth and Neonatal Death Society (SANDS) provides support for bereaved parents, and information for professionals. The parents need the chance to grieve when a miscarriage or a stillbirth occurs. The importance of rites of passage is now recognised and parents are encouraged to collect momentos of the infant and to arrange a funeral ceremony. Members of the primary health care team can ensure that patients receive appropriate support and counselling after a miscarriage[19].

Hysterectomy

The reaction of a woman after hysterectomy may range from relief at the end of miserable symptoms and the fear of pregnancy, to severe depression and grief at the supposed loss of her feminity. A practice nurse can help a patient to express her feelings. Appropriate support and counselling can be offered. The Women's Health and Reproductive Rights Information Centre has produced a booklet about hysterectomy and provides information about a national network of hysterectomy support groups[20].

A patient who has had a hysterectomy because of a malignancy will continue to need regular vaginal vault smears. Pre-menopausal women whose ovaries are removed require immediate hormone replacement therapy to prevent the effects of a sudden menopause[21]. Moreover, 24% of women with intact ovaries are likely to experience ovarian failure within two years of hysterctomy[22].

The menopause

The menopause marks the end of fertility for women as the ovaries cease to function. The decrease in oestrogen production causes physical and emotional changes, although the type and severity of symptoms can vary from one woman to another. Common symptoms include: hot flushes and night sweats. The temperature regulating centre in the hypothalamus is believed to be stimulated by the increased production of gonadotrophic hormones in response to the reduced oestrogen in the circulation. Vaginal dryness and atrophy are also caused by the lack of oestrogen.

Depression, irritability and lack of concentration are other common complaints, but caution should prevail before attributing every problem to the menopause. Unsatisfactory marital relationships, children leaving home, business worries, or unfulfilled ambitions can also lead to depression and sexual difficulties in middle age. A thorough history and medical examination is needed for each patient.

The longer term effects of the menopause include an increased risk of coronary heart disease and osteoporosis. Practice nurses are able to help women at the menopause by:

- listening to their concerns,
- providing factual information about the menopause and the treatments available,

- assessing their general health and risk factors for heart disease and osteoporosis,
- referring them to the doctor for medical assessment and treatment,
- monitoring the effects of treatment.

The management of menopausal symptoms

Practice nurses should be aware of the treatments available and encourage patients to consult their doctor when necessary. The available treatments include:

- *Local* – to relieve vaginal dryness and dyspareunia
    (a) vaginal lubricants, e.g. *KY jelly*
    (b) vaginal rehydrating gel, e.g. *Replens*
    (c) oestadiol cream, e.g. *Ortho-dinoestrol.*
- *Systemic* – for the relief of symptoms or the long-term prevention of osteoporosis and CHD
    (a) hormone replacement therapy – tablets, patches or implants
    (b) synthetic steroids – tibolone (*Livial*).

Hormone replacement therapy (HRT)

Practice nurses who advise patients about the menopause need to be familiar with the arguments for and against HRT. The proponents claim that because in evolutionary terms women were not designed to live much beyond the child-bearing years, HRT is needed to protect them from the problems associated with longevity[23]. The opposing view is that the normal menopause has been unnecessarily medicalised[24]. Also that there are far less complaints of menopausal symptoms in cultures where women gain status once they are no longer sullied by menstruation[25]. An open mind is needed, and a willingness to keep up-to-date with research into the subject. HRT can relieve many of the distressing symptoms of the menopause, but there can be side-effects. Therefore patients need careful selection and regular monitoring. Undiagnosed vaginal bleeding, pregnancy, breast or endometrial cancer are absolute contraindications to oestrogen replacement. There is less certainty about relative contraindications such as: previous CVS disease, hypertension, liver disease, diabetes, fibroids or endometriosis[26].

Patients who have had a hysterectomy can have varying strengths of oestrogen replacement alone:

- *Oral:*   *Premarin* tablets (conjugated oestrogens)
                          Climaval tablets (oestadiol)

Progynova tablets (oestradiol)
- *Transdermal:*   *Estraderm* patches (oestradiol)
Evorel patches (oestradiol)

Women who still have a uterus must also take progestogens for part of the month to oppose the proliferation of the endometrium, which can lead to endometrial cancer. Some women who object to having a monthly bleed may prefer tibolone (Livial), but this is contraindicated until one year after the last menstrual period. Examples of combined HRT preparations include:

- *Oral:*   *Prempak* C tablets (conjugated oestrogens/norgestrel)
Cyclo-Progynova (oestradiol/norgestel)
Nuvelle tablets (oestradiol/norgestel)
Climagest tablets (oestradiol/norethisterone)
Menophase tablets (mestranol/norethisterone)
Trisequens tablets (oestradiol/oestriol/norethisterone)
- *Transdermal:*   *Estrapak* patches (oestradiol)
+ tablets (norethisterone)
Estracombi patches (oestradiol)
+ double patches (oestradiol/norethisterone)

The oestrogen tablets or patches are used alone for the first part of the month, and in combination with the progestogen for the latter part. The preparations are used continuously without a break and a bleed usually occurs in the last week of each course. The progestogens can produce unwanted effects such as weight gain, bloating or mood changes. Patients may be tempted to skip the progestogen tablets unless they understand their importance. Transdermal patches release quantities of hormone through the skin to maintain the pre-menopausal blood levels. The patch is applied below the waist to the abdomen, buttock or upper thigh and left in place for three to four days. It should then be changed, using a fresh patch on a different site. Skin irritation can be reduced by waving the patch in the air before applying it, to evaporate the alcohol in the adhesive. Patches must not be applied to the breasts.

Slow release hormone implants can be introduced into the abdominal wall through a trochar. Implants need to be renewed about every six months, but some patients experience menopausal symptoms while their blood levels of oestrogen are still high. HRT injections are not available in the UK but sometimes patients will bring them from other countries and request their administration.

Osteoporosis

Lack of oestrogen affects the density of bone; with the consequent risk of fractures of the hip, wrist and spine in later life. Early menopause or a history of infrequent periods are particular risk factors, but men as well as women can develop osteoporosis. Other factors known to contribute to osteoporosis include:

- heavy smoking
- long-term corticosteroid use.
- high alcohol intake
- physical inactivity
- malnutrition
- family history of osteoporosis.

Bladder problems

Women of all ages may experience problems with the urinary bladder. A sympathetic practice nurse can help them to understand and deal with the problem or to consult the GP when necessary. The start of sexual activity or the atrophic changes after the menopause can both contribute to cystitis. (See Chapter 8).

Incontinence of urine

The control of bladder function depends on:

- intact neurological pathways
- competent pelvic muscles
- the ability to get to the toilet in time.

An assessment of the patient should include urinalysis to exclude an infection or diabetes, and a full history to identify the factors contributing to incontinence. Urodynamic studies may be arranged for patients with severe problems. Childbirth, obesity, lack of exercise and pelvic surgery can all weaken the muscles of the pelvic floor. Chronic constipation can create pressure on the bladder, and diuretics pose a particular problem for elderly people, especially when their mobility is restricted.

The GP or practice nurse can make referrals as appropriate to the district nurse, physiotherapist, occupational therapist or local continence adviser. Prime consideration should be given to helping incontinent patients to preserve their dignity. Regaining a normal weight and regular pelvic floor exercises can help patients with stress incontinence. The exercises involve tightening the muscles around the anus as if trying to avoid passing wind, and around the urethra is if trying to stop the stream of urine. This can be learnt by actually stopping the stream while emptying the bladder. Instruction leaflets can be obtained from the health promotion department, or from the Continence Foundation[27].

Information for patients

Leaflets and fact sheets are available on a wide range of topics, but patients may be too embarrassed to pick some of them up in public. Careful attention should be given to siting information in appropriate places about continence services, family planning, or sexually transmitted disease clinics.

Suggestions for evaluation and research

- Compile standards of care for nurse involvement in women's health care in your practice:
  (a) Are you able to meet all those standards?
  (b) If not, what education or resources are needed?
  (c) How do you know if the patients are satisfied with the service provided?
- Review the literature you provide for women patients:
  (a) Is it up-to-date?
  (b) Is it biased in favour of any particular product?
  (c) Is it relevant to people from different cultures?
- Audit the records of all the women age 40–55 registered with the practice:
  (a) How many have had a hysterectomy?
  (b) How many of those women have been offered or are receiving HRT?
  (c) How often is their treatment reviewed?
- Devise a confidential patient questionnaire to discover how many patients have any degree of urinary incontinence, and how it affects their lives. What help could be offered to deal with the problems identified?

References

1. Atkin, K., Lunt, W., Parker, G. and Hirst, M. (1993) *Nurses Count: A National Census of Practice Nurses*, SPRU, University of York.
2. Mathieson, E. (1991) A question of gender; *Nursing Times*, **87**, 13 February: 31–32.
3. Shreeve, C. (1992) *Premenstrual Syndrome – Curing the Real Curse*: 32–33. Thorsons, London.
4. Charny, M.C. and Farrow, S.C. (1987) Who is using cervical screening services? *Health Trends*; **19**(4): 3–5.
5. Royal College of Nursing (1994) Cervical Screening Guidelines for good practice; *Issues in Nursing and Health No. 28* RCN, London.
6. Hopwood, J., *Background to Cervical Cytology Reports*. Schering Healthcare, Sussex.
7. Winthrop Laboratories, *The Abnormal Smear*, Winthrop Practitioner Services.
8. Chamberlain, J., Moss, S.M., Kirkpatrick, A.E., Michell, M. and John, L. (1993) NHS breast screening programme results to 1991–2; *British Medical Journal*, **307**: 353–356.
9. MRC Vitamin Study Research Group (1991) Prevention of neural tube defects: results of the Medical Research Council vitamin study; *Lancet*, **338**: 131–137.
10. DOH, Welsh Office, Scottish Office Home and Health Department (1992) *Immunisation against Infectious Disease*: paragraph 11.5. HMSO.
11. Pochin, E.E. (1988) Radiation and mental retardation, *British Medical Journal*, **297**(16): 153–154.
12. Great Britain, Parliament (1990) Human Fertilisation and Embryology Act 1990, HMSO.
13. Health Education Authority (1993) *The New Pregnancy Book*, HEA, London.
14. Central Office of Information (1992) *A Guide to Maternity Benefits – Statutory Maternity Pay and Maternity Allowance*, Leaflet NI 17A, Benefits Agency.
15. News analysis (1993) Smoking in pregnancy: the facts; *Healthlines*, May 1993, HEA.
16. Waterson, J. (1985) Alcohol and pregnancy; *Nursing Times*, **81**, 28 August: 38–40.
17. Jones, D. (1990) Foodborne listeriosis; *Lancet*, **336**: 1171–1174.
18. Chief Medical Officer and Chief Nursing Officer (1993) Letter; *Vitamin A and Pregnancy*, PL/CMO (93)15, PL/CNO(93)7, Department of Health, London.
19. Jones, A. and Jones, K. (1990) Support for parents after a child's death; *Nursing Standard*, 4(46): 32–35.
20. Duin, N. and Savage, W. (1991) *Hysterectomy*, Women's Health and Reproductive Rights Information Centre, London.

21. Seeley, T. (1992) Oestrogen replacement after hysterectomy; *British Medical Journal*, **305**: 811–812.
22. Siddle, N., Sarrell, P. and Whitehead, M. (1987) The effects of hysterectomy on the age at ovarian failure: identification of a sub-group of women with premature loss of ovarian function and literature review; *Fertility and Sterility*, **47**: 94–100.
23. Belchetz, P. (1989) Hormone replacement therapy: deserves wider use; *British Medical Journal*, **298**: 1467–1468.
24. McCarthy, H. (1991) A patch too far? *Practice Nurse*, **6**: 304–305.
25. Greer, G. (1991) *The Change: Women, Ageing and the Menopause*. Hamish Hamilton.
26. Wilkes, H.C., Meade, T.W. (1991) Hormone replacement therapy in general practice; *British Medical Journal*, **302**: 1317–1320.
27. The Continence Foundation (1993) *Pelvic Floor Exercises*. CF, London.

Further reading

Health Education Authority (1993) *Approaching Parenthood – a Resource for Parent Education*. HEA, London.
Hanna, L. and Elliott, P. (1987) *Infertility and In Vitro Fertilisation*, BMA, London.
Stillbirth and Neonatal Death Society (1991) *Miscarriage, Stillbirth and Neonatal Death – Guidance for Professionals*, SANDS, London.
SANDS (1992) *A Dignified Ending: recommendations for good practice in the disposal of the bodies and remains of babies born dead before the legal age of viability*, SANDS, London.
National Osteoporosis Society (1990) *The New Approach to Osteoporosis – A Guide for General Practitioners*, NOS, Bath.
Ashworth, P.D. and Hagan, M.T. (1993) The meaning of incontinence: a qualitative study of non-geriatric urinary incontinence sufferers; *Journal of Advanced Nursing*, **18**: 1401–1407.

Useful addresses

Women's Health and Reproductive Rights Information Centre
52 Featherstone Street, London EC1Y 8RT.
Telephone 071-251 6580.

BACUP
(advice and counselling for patients with cancer and their families).
3 Bath Place, Rivington Street, London EC2A 3JR.
Telephone Freephone 0800–181199.

National Association for the Childless
318 Summer Lane, Birmingham B19 3RL.

Stillbirth and Neonatal Death Society
28 Portland Place, London W1N 4DE.
Telephone 071-436 5881.

Hysterectomy Support Group
The Venture, Green Lane, Upton, Huntingdon, Cambs PE17 5YE.

National Osteoporosis Society
PO Box 10, Radstock, Bath BA3 3YB.

Continence Foundation
The Basement, 2 Doughty Street, London WC1N 2PH.
Telephone Helpline (Mon–Fri 2–7 pm) 091-2130050.

Chapter 14
Mental Health

Holistic care grew from the recognition that physical, mental, social and spiritual well-being are all closely interlinked[1]. Project 2000 and post-registration nursing courses place emphasis on caring for the whole person within the community. Mental health nursing has always been a separate specialty, and a small proportion only of practice nurses have been educated as mental health nurses[2]. The pace and competitiveness of modern life means that more people are seeking help for stress-related illnesses; while at the same time, the closure of psychiatric institutions has shifted the focus of mental health care to the community. The staff in general practice must be able to contribute to new flexible mental health services.

The development of mental health services

Mentally ill people in the eighteenth century, whose families could not afford to confine them in private madhouses, usually ended up in prison or the workhouse. During the nineteenth century the state assumed responsibility for the care of 'lunatics' by building huge county asylums in sparsely populated areas. Social reformers campaigned for more humane treatment of the inmates.

The asylums continued to expand during the first quarter of this century but there was also a move towards alternative management. Voluntary patients and out-patients began to be treated. The county asylums came under the control of the regional hospital boards when the NHS was founded, but the provision of after-care was in the hands of the local authorities.

The development of phenothiazine drugs in the 1950s and 1960s revolutionised the treatment of patients with schizophrenia, and reduced the time they needed to be in hospital. A series of scandals, enquiries and reports brought the services for mentally ill and mentally handicapped people into public focus in the 1960s and 1970s[3,4]. At the same time there was a growth in new care facilities: day centres, hostels, and psychiatric units in general hospitals. Community psychiatric nurses grew in numbers and the first CPN post-registration course began in 1974.

The move towards care in the community led to the National Health Service and Community Care Act (1990). The closure of the Victorian institutions, which had begun in the preceeding decades, was not matched by adequate facilities for community care[5]. There were success stories of people rehabilitated after years of confinement[6]; but a huge burden was also placed on some families and carers[7]. The acute psychiatric units in some inner city areas were unable to cope adequately with the demand for acute admissions[8].

At the same time the government set targets for reducing suicide and mental illness[9]; even though high levels of unemployment, home-lessness, or drug addiction were creating negative influences on the mental and physical health of millions of people[10].

At the present time there is a need for more resources for:

- the promotion of mental health,
- the recognition and treatment of mental illness,
- social support and care for patients with mental illness and their carers,
- acute services for crisis intervention.

A mental nursing qualification can be very useful in general practice. In-house training, or attendance at mental health study days may be appropriate for other nurses. The CPN is a valuable resource for information. Depending on her/his previous experience and training, a practice nurse might be involved in these issues in some of the ways described below.

The promotion of mental health

Regular sleep, exercise, healthy food, and secure relationships – all contribute to a sense of well-being. Nurses can provide practical help and advice as required on healthy living, and also contribute to community initiatives to deter people of all ages from substance abuse.

Grief is a natural process in response to a loss, but it can turn into an abnormal reaction if it is not faced and worked through. Bereavement counselling or support groups may be needed to help a patient to deal with grief successfully. Hospices usually run training programmes on bereavement for nurses. People need a chance to talk about the intense emotional and physical feelings they experience. Sometimes, when a person has died suddenly, the one left behind is burdened by a lot of things unsaid; or words spoken in haste, which are regretted. Some people can be comforted by writing a letter to the deceased expressing those thoughts. Support groups are available in some areas for people bereaved in particular circumstances – parents who lose children, or those bereaved through violence or major disasters.

The difficulties of modern living, relationship problems, or being the victim of crime, can all cause their own problems. Recognition and acknowledgement of their existence can be the first step; so that help can be provided before a person's mental health is seriously affected.

The recognition and treatment of mental illness

Depression can sometimes be overlooked in a patient who presents multiple physical symptoms. A nurse who suspects a patient has depression may feel able to explore the issue, but in any case should refer him/her to the general practitioner.

Short-term memory problems can alert the staff to a patient's impaired mental function when he/she telephones repeatedly to ask the same questions. Many patients are aware of their memory loss and become anxious about the future. They need to be able to talk about their fears. Referral can be made to specialised memory clinics, where they exist.

Practice nurses may be required to administer regular phenothiazine injections to patients with psychotic illnesses. An understanding of the possible side-effects of the medication is required (see below). Drug treatments need to well-monitored. Blood tests are required to maintain the optimum treatment level and avoid toxicity with some drugs.

Patients with mental illness who request repeat prescriptions inappropriately may be missing medication, taking too much, or stockpiling it. The GP should be informed if this ever becomes apparent to a nurse.

The social support and care for mentally ill patients and their carers

A practice nurse might communicate with the community psychiatric nurse on the progress of a patient attending the surgery. This may be to ask for details of any previous history, or to discuss a perceived change in the patient's behaviour.

Carers may be under strain and require a chance to express their feelings, or need help to get respite care arranged. The social services are responsible for providing a case manager if a patient requires long-term community care. Supervision orders can be made for patients who could become violent to themselves or other people[11].

At times a clash of interests can occur between mental health workers and the general practice. For example, the desire of care workers to empower their clients to live independently can result in disruption in the practice when mentally ill patients, or people with learning difficulties, arrive unexpectedly and demand immediate prescriptions, or to see the doctor or nurse. Some of the patients may have a limited understanding of time or be unable to keep appointments; others may lack patience and want instant attention. Most of the difficulties can be resolved by discussion and compromise if meetings are arranged with the patients and care workers.

Acute services for crisis intervention

When a patient is well-known to a practice, the nurse may recognise when a patient's mood or behaviour has altered. A prompt referral to the GP for review may prevent a further deterioration.

When a crisis does occur, a crisis intervention team from the hospital mental health unit may be able to provide an early intensive input within the patient's home. However, sometimes a patient will need acute admission to hospital. If the patient does not accept voluntary admission, compulsory admission is permitted under the Mental Health Act (1983) if he/she is considered to be a danger to him/herself or others[12]. Serious efforts are made to safeguard the civil liberties of such patients. The compulsory detention, with which GPs are most likely to be involved, under the Mental Health Act(1983) are:

- *Section 2 – allows compulsory admission for assessment for up to 28 days.*
  The application can be from the nearest relative, or an approved social worker, and there must be a written recommendation by two medical practitioners.
- *Section 3 – allows compulsory admission for treatment for a maximum of six months.*
  The application can be made by the nearest relative or an approved social worker (with the agreement of the nearest relative), and there must be a written recommendation by two medical practitioners.
- *Section 4 – allows emergency admission for 72 hours for assessment.*
  Application by the nearest relative or an approved social worker, with written recommendation by one doctor.

There are some variations in the mental health legislation for Scotland and N. Ireland.

Dealing with aggression and violence

People who are aggressive or violent are not necessarily mentally ill, but mental illness can sometimes manifest itself this way. Patients who are very anxious or who have never learned to control their emotions can become abusive if they have to wait to see a doctor. Others can become violent under the influence of alcohol or drugs. Practice nurses and receptionists may be in the front line. 'Prevention is better than cure', and the time to consider staff safety is before an incident occurs.

Risk assessment

A survey of the practice layout and work arrangements should reveal anything which makes the staff vulnerable. Safety features should be incorporated in the design of practices and health centres. There must be a way of getting help quickly; as well as a practice policy specifying the action to be taken if an aggressive incident occurs. A receptionist or nurse could be at risk while alone in the building if members of the public have access. In such instances the front door should be kept locked, and a safety chain put on before opening the door to callers.

Nurses and doctors who undertake home visits need to consider the potential dangers and take appropriate precautions:

- Make sure someone knows where you have gone and when to expect you back. A mobile telephone can be a good investment.
- Get all the relevant details of the patient's history and social situation beforehand.
- Report back after finishing the visits, or if delayed.
- Arrange a coded message to be used if help is needed. All the staff must understand the significance of such a message.
- Be aware of any danger signs – abusive language, strange behaviour, dangerous weapons on view. Do not enter if in doubt.
- Carry a personal alarm to attract attention if attacked in the street.
- Report any worrying incidents to colleagues, and the police (if appropriate).

Staff training can be organised in ways of dealing with difficult situations. The CPN may be willing to teach some methods for avoiding confrontations, and the police will give instruction in self-preservation.

Some things to consider for avoiding incidents:

- *Keep patients informed* of what is happening and offer alternative choices if a delay is inevitable.
- *Listen to what the patient is saying.* Allow frustrations to be expressed, without responding defensively. Acknowledge any legitimate cause for complaint and apologise.
- *Avoid confrontation.* Use a quiet, calm voice even if the patient is shouting. Adopt a non-threatening posture and do not fold the arms, as this can be interpreted as aggression. Avoid staring; this can be interpreted as provocation. Try to get the patient away from others in the vicinity.
- *Get someone to phone for the police* if a situation looks likely to get out of control.
- *Avoid being injured.* Stand just out of arm's reach, with the body at an angle so it is not square-on to the patient. Have one foot slightly in front of the other to allow the body to tilt backwards. Endeavour to have a clear escape route and keep an eye out for anything which the patient might use as a weapon. Politely ask the patient to put down a weapon being held. Look out for something to use as a shield in case it is needed. Don't intervene if the patient breaks something; this can be a way of 'letting off steam'[13].

Reporting incidents

A report should be made of any aggressive incidents. Verbal abuse should be recorded in the patient's records. Any violence, or injuries inflicted must be documented in an incident report, as well as in the records. Staff who have been subjected to aggression require a chance to discuss their feelings about the incident. Professional counselling may be needed in some instances.

Helping patients with mental health problems

It is beyond the scope of this book to discuss all the ways mental illness might be classified. This chapter deals mainly with the situations which practice nurses are most likely to encounter.

Stress

The word *stress* is often used nowadays to indicate any situation in which a person feels unable to cope with life's demands. The fear of chronic habituation to tranquillisers has led to the search for safer ways to help. The distressing symptoms derive from biological reactions which evolved to help our primitive ancestors to survive in the face of danger – the 'fight or flight' response. There is usually a balance within the body between the parasympathetic and sympathetic nervous activity; but the outpouring of adrenaline in response to perceived danger stimulates the sympathetic nervous system. This is predominantly responsible for the effects associated with stress (see Fig. 14.1). At the same time, parasympathetic stimulation of the gastro-intestinal tract can also result in nausea and diarrhoea.

A certain level of arousal is needed for normal social functioning and to avoid accidents. Long periods of understimulation will result in boredom, loss of concentration and apathy. Prolonged overstimulation can cause a breakdown in the body's ability to adapt, resulting in physical or mental illness. There may be a genetic link with the way individuals react to stress[14]. Something which might overwhelm one person, could seem an exciting challenge to another. Single major stressors such as bereavement, divorce or business failure may precipitate a stress-related illness; or there may be multiple small events until a crisis point is reached.

Post-traumatic stress disorder has recently been recognised as a consequence of major disasters[15]. Special counselling is provided for

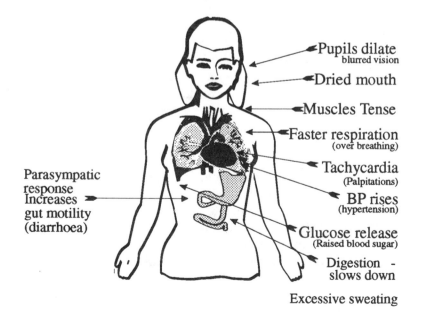

Fig. 14.1 The effects of stress on the body.

survivors and families following these events. Many of the unfortunate young soldiers shot for desertion during the First World War were probably suffering from this condition[16].

Patients may consult the GP with a variety of symptoms which are ultimately attributed to stress: insomnia, depression, constant tiredness, panic attacks, muscular pains, indigestion, skin disorders, and head-aches. Counselling can help a patient to identify the problems, and find the solutions. A situation incapable of a solution is not really a problem – it's a fact of life. Sometimes people need help to differentiate between the two, and to learn to live with the facts of life.

Depending on the circumstances, various strategies or support agencies might be appropriate:

- Developing self-awareness. Helping the individual to understand his/ her behaviour. Learning to express powerful feelings – anger, grief, fear, or guilt and to accept the need for other people.
- *Assertiveness training.* Learning to express personal needs or to refuse requests without giving offence. Assertive parenting can minimise the conflict with children.
- *Dealing with relationships:*
    (a) *Children.* The health visitor can often advise on assertive parenting skills, to minimise the conflict with children. Childcare arrangements may allow parents some freedom. Referral for family therapy may be needed for disturbed children.
    (b) *Partners.* Advice about birth control can help in limiting the size of families. Counselling services such as Relate, or some churches, can help with relationship problems. Gay and lesbian self-help groups can provide specific support. Bereavement counselling services are available for bereaved partners.
    (c) *Dependants.* Community nurses and social services can provide help for carers. Respite care can be arranged, and carers' associations can provide practical and emotional help.
- *Finance.* Learning to live within an income, or deal with debts. Citizens Advice Bureaux will advise. Ensure benefits are being claimed (if applicable). Leaflets about entitlement can be obtained from main post offices and social security offices.
- *Time-management.* Learning to identify priorities for action, and to make time for recreation and rest.
- *Enjoying work.* Learning to delegate, or even looking for alternative work if not happy.
- *Finding alternatives.* Unemployment, retirement, or children leav-

ing home can leave a big gap in a patient's life. Part-time work, voluntary work, a hobby or study might provide an answer.

- *Relaxation.* Learning to counteract the physical effects of stress by: physical exercise, yoga, therapeutic massage, aromatherapy, or relaxation exercises and tapes.

Disorders of affect (disturbance of mood)

Depression

Most people experience a feeling of depression at some time. Depression is a disorder of affect in which the mood is flattened. The sufferer may report a loss of appetite, sleep disturbance – especially early morning wakening, fatigue, lethargy and lack of concentration. There may be disordered thought processes, agitation and anxiety, or feelings of hopelessness which can lead to suicide. Some people indulge in binge-eating when depressed. The severity of the symptoms experienced can vary and the underlying problem may not always be recognised. The Defeat Depression Campaign was launched in 1992 by the Royal College of General Practitioners and the Royal College of Psychiatrists, to educate the public and professionals and to help members of the PHCT to detect depression and to support patients being treated for the condition.

Depression may develop as a reaction to a major life event – bereavement, illness, or loss of employment, and it can sometimes seem easier to relate to the feelings of a person with this type of reactive depression, than to understand a patient with endogenous depression which develops for no apparent reason.

Treatment of depression

Antidepressant drugs might be needed in order to lift the black mood, and counselling may help patients to develop a more positive view of life and their ability to control events.

Most antidepressants prescribed in general practice belong to the tricyclic group (e.g. amitriptyline). There are many variations of these; some of which are slow release preparations which only need to be taken once a day. They have a number of features in common:

- They tend to be sedative, and potentiate alcohol. The sedative effects are less marked the longer they are taken.
- They are lethal in overdose, especially if taken with alcohol.
- Any beneficial antidepressant effects are unlikely to be felt in less

than two or three weeks from starting treatment and patients should be encouraged to persevere with the treatment even if they are feeling no better.

● They may have other side-effects like blurred vision or dry mouth, which may cause a patient to stop taking them.

Monoamine oxidase inhibitors (MOAIs) are a group of antidepressants used in certain types of depression and phobic states. Great care needs to be exercised with this group as they interact with many other drugs and foodstuffs. All patients taking MAOIs must be warned of this and given written instructions stating:

● The drug should be used with care.
● No other drugs, including aspirin, should be taken without discussion with the doctor.
● Foodstuffs containing tyramine will react with MAOIs to produce a severe rise in blood pressure. These foods include cheese, Bovril and Marmite. (See *MIMS* for the complete list.)
● 5HT reuptake inhibitors (e.g. fluoxetine hydrochloride) are a newer group of antidepressant drugs which have a less sedative effect. They may cause gastro-intestinal upsets or more disturbing neurological side-effects. Consult the *British National Formulary* for details of the action and contraindications and side-effects of these and other types of anti-depressant drugs.

Mania

Mania has the opposite effect to depression. The patient is over-energetic and enthusiastic, with rapid speech and thought processes. Grandiose schemes, flights of fancy, and wild financial expenditure can cause great distress to the families affected. Sometimes the mania alternates with bouts of black depression, with periods of 'normality' in between.

Treatment of mania

Lithium carbonate is most commonly used to control the mood swings. Blood levels need to be taken regularly to adjust the dose if it is approaching the toxic level. The blood sample should be obtained just before the next dose is due, so the residual blood level is established. The time elapsed since the last dose should be recorded on the pathology request form.

Psychotic disorders

Patients with psychotic disorders have a different way of viewing themselves and the world. Their behaviour may endanger themselves and cause distress or fear to others. Help is then needed to prevent injury and restore the patient's ability to function within society. The disordered thought processes and behaviour can be manifested in many ways.

Schizophrenia

This is a name which covers a range of conditions. The speech pattern may be bizarre; emotions may either be dulled or wholly inappropriate to the situation; the person may be withdrawn or self-absorbed or behave in ways which seem incongruous in their context; normal tasks cannot be completed. Hallucinations can lead to violence in response to instructions from 'the voices'. There may be delusions of grandeur or of persecution.

Treatment

Many patients receive long-acting anti-psychotic drugs, e.g. fluphenazine (*Modecate*) and flupenthixol (*Depixol*). There should be a protocol and standards of care written for practice nurses who administer depot injections covering:

Nurse education: a practice nurse requires an understanding of the nature, recognition and treatment of schizophrenia, including the side-effects of the medication.

Recall system: patients who do not keep their appointment must be followed up quickly and the GP informed. By the nature of the disorder, once a patient misses the treatment, he/she will not recognise the need for the medication as a relapse occurs.

Authorisation: there must be a written prescription signed by the GP or hospital psychiatrist for each patient. The dose may need to be adjusted periodically, and it is important that the nurse is aware of any changes.

Stocks: drugs for injection can either be obtained by each patient on individual prescriptions; or be purchased by the practice and reimbursement claimed for the prescriptions monthly.

Administration: patients with mental illness should have the same well-person screening and the treatment of physical symptoms, as other patients. Depot injections should not be given in pregnancy.

A test dose should be administered in case of adverse reactions. The lowest dose of the drug available should be used the first time. The medication should be administered by deep I/M injection into the upper, outer quadrant of the buttock.

At subsequent visits the patient should be asked how the injection is helping and if it is causing any problems. Some patients gain weight with the medication. Parkinsonism is a side-effect of phenothiazine drugs, due to their dopamine blocking activity. The nurse should look for signs of tremor or tardive dyskinesia. The GP may need to reduce the dose of depot medication or prescribe anti-Parkinson's drugs to counteract the side-effects.

The time intervals between injections can vary. Three weekly is the usual time, but it can range from weekly to monthly, according to the patient's needs. The patient should be encouraged to make the next appointment before leaving. Reminders may need to be given to patients who are likely to forget to attend.

Annual blood tests for urea and electrolytes and liver function tests may be requested to detect any dysfunction.

Records: the injections given must be documented appropriately (see Chapter 5).

Dementia

Loss of memory for recent events is an early sign of dementia. An inability to perform everyday tasks or to interact socially can follow as all the higher mental functions become impaired. The degree and speed of impairment can vary between patients. The diagnosis is made clinically, once all the other causes of confusion have been eliminated.

Looking after a person with dementia can pose enormous strains on the care-givers. Care in the community should not be achieved at the expense of the physical and mental health of carers. Practice nurses can offer a friendly ear as well as ensuring that carers receive information about all the services and support available. Many local authorities now produce a directory of local services. The Alzheimer's Disease Society provides information and practical support. Many of the volunteers have had personal experiences of caring for a relative with dementia. There are also support groups for people with other sorts of dementia, for example, Parkinson's disease, Huntingdon's chorea, or AIDS.

A balance needs to be maintained between helping people with dementia as their faculties decline, and making them unnecessarily dependent. Carers need help to identify realistic expectations and to take some risks.

Substance abuse

Drugs have been used for their mind-altering properties for millennia.

Tobacco and alcohol provide our Inland Revenue with vast sums of money every year, which makes a mockery of the funds put into health promotion. Drug dealing is the only growth industry in some inner-city areas.

Dependence on an addictive substance occurs when a person cannot cope without it. Physical or psychological dependance eventually causes the body to develop tolerance to the substance and ever larger amounts are needed to create the same effect. Severe physical or psychological withdrawal effects are experienced if the substance is not available for any reason.

Alcohol

Alcohol in small quantities is not usually harmful, and there may even be some beneficial effects[17]. Alcohol is a central nervous system depressant, although initially it may create a sense of euphoria. Regular alcohol use can result in dependance. Deprivation of alcohol can then cause depression, anxiety, convulsions and terrifying hallucinations.

Practice nurses may identify patients who already have or are in danger of developing a dependance on alcohol. Many health promotion units organise training in counselling patients about alcohol. Patients may be reluctant to admit their actual daily consumption. *Better Living – Better Life* has a section on sensible drinking and the questions which can help to identify problem drinkers[18].

Patients who seek help for alcohol dependance may be referred for detoxification. Long-term support will be needed to cope afterwards. Alcoholics Anonymous and other self-help groups provide peer support. Al-Anon and Al-Ateen provide support for the families of problem drinkers.

Drug abuse

The use of drugs and other substances depends to a certain extent on both their availability and on social pressures. Now that smoking is less socially acceptable, many people find themselves outnumbered at social gatherings. On the other hand, the peer pressure to experiment with drugs, alcohol or tobacco can be hard for young people to resist, and solvents are readily available.

Heroin

Heroin is an opium derivative with powerful analgesic properties which can also induce a sence of euphoria. The drug may be injected or inhaled ('snorted'). Tolerance quickly develops, so larger quantities are required. Self-neglect, weight loss, anaemia and infections can follow. The absence of quality control with illegal drugs means that they often contain impurities. However, accidental overdosing with unusually pure forms can result in death. Abscesses and septicaemia can develop from dirty needles, and users who share equipment or who prostitute themselves to get money for drugs, are at risk of developing and spreading HIV infection and hepatitis.

Cocaine

Cocaine is a powerful stimulant derived from the coca plant which creates a psychological dependance. It is usually sniffed or smoked. Crack, a highly addictive concentrated form of cocaine is now freely available and posing a new problem for the law enforcement agencies.

Amphetamines

Amphetamines ('uppers') are stimulants which create a feeling of increased energy and excitement. The user is restless and overactive but exhaustion can occur later, especially if the drug is injected ('mainlining speed'). Sedatives ('downers') may be taken in order to sleep.

Hallucinogens

Hallucinogens are taken for their mind-altering effects. Some are more dangerous than others. They include cannabis and LSD.

Cannabis

Cannabis is obtained in dried leaf form, as resin, or a concentrated oil. It is usually smoked but can be ingested with food. It can cause a mild euphoria and sense of well-being. It is not addictive but association with the illegal drug culture can encourage the move to more harmful substances. Some dealers have been known to mix crack with cannabis in order to create addiction[19].

Lysergic acid diethylamide (LSD)

LSD ('acid') causes hallucinating effects which last for up to 12 hours ('a trip'). During that time the user may have sense of disassociation from the body and be at risk from dangerous behaviour like trying to fly. LSD tablets are relatively cheap and freely available at acid house parties and raves.

Solvents

The fumes from any volatile substance – glue, anti-freeze, lighter fuel, nail varnish remover, or aerosol propellants, can be inhaled from a plastic bag. The effects produced can look similar to intoxication with alcohol, but redness around the mouth, and running eyes and nose can be a give-away. There may be a history of poor school performance and truancy. Respiratory and renal failure can be caused by solvent abuse, as well as accidents due to dangerous behaviour; or death from asphyxia or inhaled vomit.

Substance abuse is a major current health problem. Practice nurses can provide information about addictive substances to parents and young people in the practice. A nurse may detect signs of possible solvent abuse, or note needle marks when taking a blood pressure or treating a wound. Patients may attend the surgery with physical complaints of weight-loss, fatigue, gastric problems, blackouts, or accidents. There may also be reports of relationship problems, altered behaviour, absenteeism, financial problems, or self-neglect. Family members of people who misuse substances may be seen with frequent minor ailments which mask the true cause of their distress.

Eating disorders

Hunger is a physiological drive to eat in response to the body's needs for energy and nutrients. The appetite for certain foods can be indulged, or overridden, irrespective of the feelings of hunger. Social and familial customs and beliefs associated with food can affect an individual person's eating behaviour.

Anorexia nervosa

Sufferers from anorexia nervosa have a distorted body image which makes them strive for an abnormally low weight because they mistakenly believe they are fat. Calorie intakes are strictly regulated and eating may be followed by induced vomiting. Female sufferers usually develop amenorrhoea as a result of starvation. Death can result if the process is not reversed.

Bulimia nervosa

With bulimia, periods of binge-eating are interspersed with vomiting, purging and violent exercise in an attempt to prevent weight gain. The shame and guilt associated with this loss of control reinforces the individual's poor self-image.

Practice nurses weigh patients during screening and well-person checks. Patients with anorexia nervosa may be identified by finding a very low BMI, but they are likely to deny having a problem. Patients with bulimia may have a normal weight/height ratio yet complain of being overweight. They may also have a past history of anorexia nervosa. The knuckles of patients with an eating disorder may be scarred by their teeth from persistently inducing vomiting. Referral is needed for specialised help for eating disorders.

Obesity

Obesity, defined as a BMI over 30, results from a consistent intake of more calories than the body requires for energy. The compulsion to eat can be overwhelming even when a person is unhappy with his/her size and wants to lose weight. Fortunes are spent every year on diets and 'wonder drugs'.

Genetic factors as well a learned behaviour within the family may be involved. There may also be biochemical stimuli which provoke cravings for certain foods. Inappropriate eating can also be a cover for other psychological problems[20]. The concentration on food and weight provides a way to avoid facing the deeper conflicts. Unfortunately, there is a tendency nowadays to castigate individuals who cannot stick to a healthy diet. Practice nurses can offer dietary advice and encouragement but success will not usually be sustained unless the patient can deal with the underlying problems as well.

Self awareness in the caring professions

In order to provide empathetic support and care for patients and their families, nurses and doctors have to be able to deal with their own problems as human beings. Many people in the caring professions seem to have a particular need to to be admired and respected; so emotional conflict can arise if patients appear demanding or ungrateful[21]. All the members of the primary health care team should be encouraged to explore their own feelings and motivations. A private journal or tape-recording can be a way of expressing personal feelings[22]. Co-counselling is a method whereby practitioners work in pairs to counsel each other[23]. This is probably better done with a co-counsellor unconnected with the same GP practice. Other forms of counselling should be sought if they are needed.

Suggestions for evaluation and research

- Review your professional profile:
    (a) How well equipped do you feel you are for dealing with the mental health issues encountered during your work?
    (b) Prepare learning objectives for any further training you think you need.
- Reflect on the last few encounters you have had with patients with mental illness:
    (a) How well did you communicate?
    (b) With the benefit of hindsight, would you have done anything differently?
- Audit the nursing records of patients having depot medication:
    (a) How often are physical or mental symptoms recorded?
    (b) What action was taken when those symptoms were recorded?
    (c) When was each patient last reviewed by a doctor?
- Prepare a small-scale study of the drug problem in your locality. Consider ways in which the primary health care team might target help.

References

1. Martin, J.O. (1993) 'Holism' in the discourse of nursing; *Journal of Advanced Nursing*, **18:** 1688–1695.
2. Atkin, K., Lunt, N., Parker, G. and Hirst, M. (1993) *Nurses Count: A National Census of Practice Nurses.* SPRU, University of York.
3. Robb, B. (1967) *Sans Everything, A Case to Answer.* Nelson, London.
4. Secretary of State for Social Services (1978) *Report of the Committee of Inquiry into Normansfield Hospital.* HMSO, London.
5. George, M. (1992) Home care support; *Community Outlook.* 2(2): 12–13.
6. Feature (1992) Helping in the home; *Nursing Standard*, 7(3): 20–21.
7. Nolan, M.R. and Grant, L. (1989) Addressing the needs of informal carers: a neglected area of nursing practice; *Journal of Advanced Nursing*, **14:** 950–961.
8. Darcy, P. (1994) Accountability and the mental health services; *British Journal of Nursing*, **3:** 254–255.
9. Department of Health (1992) *The Health of the Nation: A Strategy for Health in England.* HMSO, London.

10. Kammerly, R.M. and O'Connor, S. (1993) Unemployment rate as predictor of rate of psychiatric admissions; *British Medical Journal*, **307:** 1536–1539.
11. Department of Health (1994) *Guidance on the Discharge of Mentally Disordered People and their Continuing Care in the Community.* HMSO, London.
12. Great Britain, Parliament (1983) *The Mental Health Act 1983.* HMSO, London.
13. Walsh, M. (1990) *Accident and Emergency Nursing – a New Approach*; Violence and aggression: 271–276. Butterworth Heinemann, Oxford.
14. Wright, H. and Giddey, M. (1993) *Mental Health Nursing: From First Principles to Professional Practice:* 112. Chapman and Hall, London.
15. McKinley, B. and Brooks, N. (1991) Post-traumatic stress disorder explained; *Nursing Standard*, **5** (30 January): 50–51.
16. Brandon, S. (1991) The psychological aftermath of war; *British Medical Journal*, **302:** 305–306.
17. Marmot, M. and Brunner, E. (1991) Alcohol and cardiovascular disease: the status of the U shaped curve; *British Medical Journal*, **303:** 565–568.
18. DOH, General Medical Services Committee and Royal College of General Practitioners working group on Health Promotion (1993) *Better Living – Better Life.* Knowledge House, Henley on Thames.
19. Walsh, M. (1990) *Accident and Emergency Nursing* (2nd Edn): 249. Butterworth Heinnemann, Oxford.
20. Ryle, A. and Evans, C.D.H. (1991) Some meanings of body and self in eating disordered and comparison subjects; *British Journal of Medical Psychology*, **64**(3): 273–283.
21. Colman, R. (1993) Patient power; *Nursing Times*, **89**(47): 50.
22. Wright, H. and Giddey, M. (Eds) (1993) *Mental Health Nursing: From First Principles to Professional Practice:* 369. Chapman and Hall, London.
23. Woddis, C. (1987) The counsel of equals; *Openmind*, **26** (April/May): 10–11.

Further reading

Dimond, B. (1990) Legal aspects of care of the mentally disordered; *Practice Nurse*, **2:** 455–464.
Jacob, S.R. (1993) An analysis of the concept of grief; *Journal of Advanced Nursing*, **18:** 1787–1794.
Hussein Rassool, G. (1993) Nursing and substance misuse: responding to the challenge; *Journal of Advanced Nursing*, **18:** 1415–1423.
Burke, A. (1993) Ecstasy can kill; *Practice Nursing*, 21 Sept–4 Oct: 17–18.
Worden, W.J. (1983) *Grief Counselling and Grief Therapy.* Tavistock Publications, London.
Roet, B. (1987) *All in the Mind? Think Yourself Better.* Macdonald Optima, London.
Farrell, G.A. and Gray, C. (1992) *Aggression – A Nurses' Guide to Therapeutic Management.* Scutari Press, London.

Useful addresses

British Association for Counselling
1 Regent Place,
Rugby,
West Midlands, CV21 2PJ.
Telephone 0788-578328.

National Association for Mental Health (MIND)
22 Harley Street,
London W1N 2ED.

Schizophrenia Association of Great Britain,
Bryn Hyfryd,
The Crescent,
Bangor LL57 2AG.
Telephone 0248-354048.

Carers National Association
20–25 Glasshouse Yard
London EC1A 4JS
Telephone 071-480 8818

Alzheimer's Disease Society
10 Greencoat Place,
London SW1P 1PH.
Telephone 071-306 0606.

Institute for the Study of Drug Dependency
1 Hatton Place,
London EC1N 8ND.
Telephone 071-928 1211.

Re-Solv
30 High Street,
Stone,
Staffs, ST15 8AW.

Overeaters Anonymous
PO Box 19,
Stretford,
Manchester M32 9EB.
(Send sae for the address of nearest local group).

Chapter 15
Health Promotion for Patients with Chronic Diseases

The 1990 GP Contract gave an impetus to the involvement of practice nurses in chronic disease management, and nurses have proved they can work well to protocols for this purpose[1]. Asthma, diabetes and hypertension were the first conditions with which large numbers of practice nurses developed expertise, but epilepsy, skin diseases, gastro-intestinal conditions and blood disorders are ripe for more nurse involvement. No one nurse can expect to be sufficiently knowledgeable in all these subjects; yet the possiblities should not be overlooked. Many practices now employ more than one nurse, so there is nothing to stop each of them from specialising in different fields. All the practice nurse journals have regular articles on chronic disease management.

Any patient who attends a clinic at a GP surgery or health centre has a right to expect a uniformly high standard of service. The following points should be considered when writing the standards of care:

1. Aims

The aims of each clinic should be specified. Most clinics for chronic disease management will have similar aims:

- to help the patients and their families to understand the disease and take responsibility for its control,
- to minimise the number of critical incidents,
- to help the patients to lead as normal a life as possible.

2. Target groups

The target groups may be all the patients known or suspected of having a particular disease, for example all patients with asthma; or a sub-group, such as patients with non-insulin dependent diabetes.

3. Organisation

The way a clinic is to be organised, and the amount of time to be allocated to each consultation has to be decided in advance. The equipment needed and record systems have to be arranged. In order to comply with the *Code of Professional Conduct* a nurse will require the appropriate education before attempting to run a clinic. Secretarial support is necessary for contacting the patients and making appointments, so the nurse's time is used most effectively. A disease register and call/recall system is needed for each clinic (see Chapter 3).

Although the word 'clinic' is used for convenience throughout this chapter, patients do not necessarily need to be seen at special clinic times; they may be seen during normal surgery hours. Some sessions may be more convenient for the patients if arranged when other health professionals, such as a dietician and chiropodist, are working in the practice. It is preferable to have a doctor available during nurse-run clinics because a medical examination, prescription, or hospital referral may be needed.

4. Protocols for nurse-run clinics

A protocol can be tailored to minimum, moderate or maximum nursing input, in accordance with the practice nurse's knowledge and experience. Each protocol should specify the procedure to be followed at first and subsequent clinic appointments. Some sources of specimen protocols are given in the relevant sections below.

5. Outcome

The standards should specify the benefits expected for the patients, and the way the clinic will be audited.

Asthma

Asthma is an inflammatory disease of the airways characterised by narrowing of the bronchioles from:

- spasm of the smooth muscle in the walls of the bronchioles
- swelling of the mucosa
- thick mucus secretion. (See Fig. 15.1.)

The condition is intermittent and reversible; either spontaneously, or

Normal Bronchiole

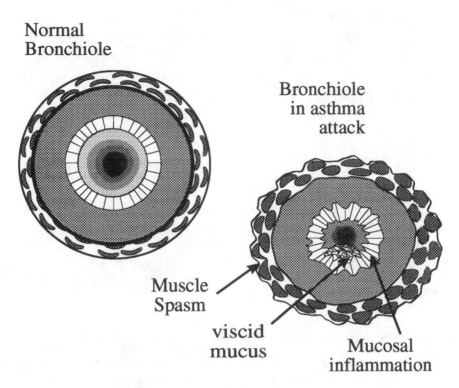

Bronchiole
in asthma
attack

Muscle
Spasm

viscid
mucus

Mucosal
inflammation

Fig. 15.1 The effects of asthma on the airway.

when the correct treatment is given. About 2000 deaths from asthma still occur annually in the UK, although this could be interpreted as a reduction in the death rate when compared with the increased incidence of asthma[2].

Incidence

In a practice with 8000 patients, 400 of them can be expected to have asthma. Children have the highest incidence of asthma but the condition can begin at any age. About 10–15% of children are estimated to be affected. Three-quarters of them may grow out of it, but unfortunately about 50% of those who do grow out of it can expect to get asthma again in later life[3].

Causes

The trigger factors which precipitate asthma can be allergic or non-allergic. Anyone could have an asthma attack if exposed to a large enough trigger factor. People with asthma differ in having hyper-reactive airways, which react to even small contact with triggers. Allergic triggers include: house dust mites, pollen, moulds and spores, animal dander, and chemicals. Non-allergic triggers can be: exercise, upper respiratory tract infections, cold air, cigarette smoke, and emotional stress. The common cold is a very common trigger.

The aim of treatment is to suppress the bronchial hyper-reactivity, and the key to good control lies in compliance with the treatment. A patient who feels fit and well may be reluctant to continue with preventive therapy unless its importance is fully appreciated.

Asthma treatments (refer to the *British National Formulary*)

The British Thoracic Society has issued guidelines on a step-wise approach to treatment, so that the maximum control of asthma symptoms is achieved by using the most appropriate drugs[4].

Bronchodilators

The commonly used drugs in this field are the beta$_2$ stimulants – salbutamol (*Ventolin*) and terbutaline (*Bricanyl*) which act mainly by relaxing bronchial smooth muscle; thus relieving bronchospasm. For this reason bronchodilators are called 'reliever' drugs.

Modified release theophylline preparations

Oral preparations of theophylline (e.g. *Slo-Phyllin, Uniphyllin Continus*) are bronchodilators which can be used to relieve nocturnal or early-morning asthma. The dose has to be carefully adjusted for each patient, and the same brand should be ordered each time. Generic prescribing is not appropriate for these drugs[5].

Mast cell stabilisers

Sodium cromoglycate (*Intal*) is often more effective in children than adults. It can be used as prophylaxis for allergic and exercise induced asthma, by inhibiting the release of histamine and similar substances. The treatment needs to be used regularly, even when there are no symptoms of asthma.

Corticosteroids

Patients who need to use a reliever drug more than once or twice a day usually require inhaled steroids to deal with the inflammation of the bronchial mucosa, for example beclomethasone dipropionate (*AeroBec*, *Becotide, Becloforte*) or budesonide (*Pulmicort*). Patients often have confused ideas about steroids and are reluctant to use them long-term. It is important to explain their action as '*preventers*' and to ensure patients know how to use them. Fungal infections of the mouth and throat are possible side-effects. Patients can be advised to have a drink after using the steroid inhaler. High-dose steroids should used with a spacer device.

Fluticasone propionate (*Flixotide*) is a recently introduced inhaled steroid which the manufacturers claim has a less detrimental effect on children's growth than other inhaled steroids[6].

A short course of oral steroids may be prescribed after treatment with a nebulised bronchodilator for acute asthma (see Chapter 7, *Emergency Situations*).

Occasionally patients require daily small doses of oral steroids to control chronic asthma symptoms. Patients on maintenance therapy should be given a steroid card to carry, and be warned not to stop the drugs suddenly.

Longer-acting beta$_2$ stimulant

Salmeterol (*Serevent*) is a longer-acting bronchodilator, useful in some cases for night-time and exercise-induced asthma. It should not be used as a 'reliever' drug. This type of drug has been named a '*protector*'. *Salmeterol* should be used in conjunction with other asthma therapy, and the effects closely monitored.

Delivery systems

- *metered dose inhalers* (with or without spacer devices), e.g. *Brica-nyl, Ventolin, Intal, Becotide, Pulmicort, Becloforte, Serevent* (see Fig. 15.2),
- *breath-actuated metered dose inhalers*, e.g. *Aerolin Autohaler, Intal Fisonair, Aerobec Autohaler,*
- *dry powder devices*, e.g. *Ventolin* and *Becotide Rotacaps* used with a *Rotahaler*, pre-loaded *Bricanyl* and *Pulmicort Turbohalers, Intal Spincaps* used with a *Spinhaler, Ventodisk, Becodisk* and *Serevent* disks used with a *Diskhaler*.

Nurses should familiarise themselves with the way all these devices are used. Sales representatives will supply placebo inhalers for teaching purposes.

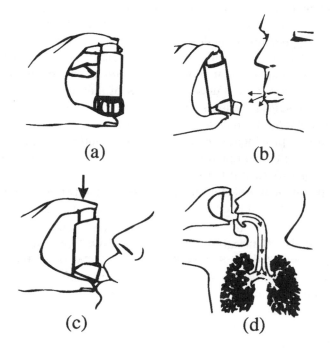

Fig. 15.2   How to use a metered dose inhaler. (a) Remove the cover from the mouthpiece. Hold the mouthpiece as illustrated and shake vigorously. (b) Breathe out slowly but no further than the end of a natural breath. (c) *Immediately* place the mouthpiece above the tongue and well into the mouth. Press the top of the canister down firmly between forefinger and thumb whilst inhaling deeply. (d) Continue inhaling to carry the spray deep into the lungs. Hold the breath for as long as it is comfortable. Release pressure on the canister, remove the inhaler from your mouth and breath out gently.

Asthma clinics

Nurse education

The Asthma Training Centre (ATC) at Stratford upon Avon organises training for practice nurses, and awards the Diploma in Asthma Care jointly with the RCGP. A distance learning package is followed by consolidation and the examination at a regional training centre. Introductory and updating sessions are also run locally by the ATC asthma trainers. The Diploma in Asthma Care attracts 24 CATS points at level 2 (see Chapter 2).

The ATC produces a newsletter for diplomates, and the asthma trainers contribute regular articles to the practice nurse journals.

Equipment

The following equipment is needed:

- scales and height chart,
- PEFR meter and mouthpiece for adults and children,
- PEFR prediction calculator or charts,
- bronchodilator for reversibility tests,
- placebo inhalers for teaching inhaler tecniques,
- explanatory booklets for adults and children,
- instruction leaflets, diagrams and peak flow diaries,
- information about voluntary organisations and other services.

Many of the asthma drug companies provide useful materials for nurses and patients. The National Asthma Campaign (NAC) publishes a range of educational booklets, and runs the Asthma Helpline which provides telephone counselling and advice. The NAC Junior Asthma Club has its own newsletter, books and comics for children.

Protocol

The Asthma Training Centre has produced guidelines for minimum, medium and maximum nurse involvement as part of the distance learning package. The RCN's *Protocols for Health Promotion Clinics* contains a sample protocol for asthma care[7].

Procedure for a first consultation

(A patient with suspected, or newly diagnosed asthma.)

History

- Past medical history: including allergies or eczema.
- Asthma history: age at onset, trigger factors, symptoms and treatments used.
- Family history: including atopic conditions.
- Social history: smoking and exercise, occupation and any relationship of the asthma to work.

Current medication

Are inhalers used?

Tests and examination

- General health assessment: to identify any risk factors and establish a baseline. (Include BP, height and weight and urinalysis.) Steroids can affect growth in children and precipitate diabetes in some patients.
- Peak expiratory flow rate (see Chapter 6). Compare with the predicted PEFR.

Diagnostic tests

(If asthma is not yet confirmed.)

- Reversibility test: record the PEFR immediately before and ten minutes after inhaling salbutamol or terbutaline. If the PEFR improves by 15% or more this is diagnostic of asthma.
- Exercise tolerance test (if appropriate for the patient): record the PEFR before and after six minutes exercise. PEFR should be recorded at five minute intervals for 15 minutes. The diagnosis of asthma will be confirmed if the peak low falls by 15% or more. Recovery may be spontaneous, but if necesary an inhaled bronchodilator can be used.
- Serial peak flow readings: ask the patient to keep a diary of twice daily readings and to record any symptoms. A 5% difference between the morning and evening reading is normal, but differences of 15% or more indicate asthma.
- Steroid trial: to see if a significant improvement is achieved, when reversibility tests have been unimpressive.

General health promotion

(See Chapter 9.)
Discuss the factors which may affect the asthma most.

Specific health promotion

- Explain the nature of asthma so that the patient can comprehend. Parents of children with asthma can have their lives severely disrupted. They need a chance to talk about their anxieties and to learn as much as possible about asthma. Asthma story books can be used for small children.
- Explain how the treatment works and how and when to use it.
- Identify the trigger factors to be avoided, e.g. smoking by parents.

- Patients and parents need to be aware of the signs of worsening asthma and when to contact the GP.
- Provide information about the voluntary societies.

Inhaler technique

Select the most suitable device and teach the parent or patient how to use it.

PEFR monitoring

Teach the patient how to monitor and record his/her peak flow at home (if able to use a peak flow meter).

Procedure for subsequent visits:

Progress

- Discuss the asthma diary and any significant entries.
- Discuss other lifestyle factors, e.g. smoking, work or schooling missed.
- Discuss any problems with the medication.

Observations

- Check the PEFR and compare with the predicted rate.
- Check the patient's inhaler technique, reteach if necessary, or consider an alternative delivery system. Give praise generously when it is due.

Education

- Ask the patient or parent to explain what he/she understands about asthma and its treatment. Correct gently any misunderstandings. It is important to be sure that the patient really has understood. What seems very basic physiology to a nurse, may be quite incomprehensible to a lay person.
- Advise about influenza immunisation each year.
- Patients who are familiar with their asthma can be given self-management cards which tell them what to do in particular circumstances. For example:

PEFR below 70%   Repeat relief treatment and double the dose of inhaled steroid.

PEFR below 50%   Start course of oral steroids and call the GP or asthma clinic nurse.

Records

Patients who are able to do so should keep their own asthma diaries. The National Asthma Campaign produces treatment cards for patients to carry, and for children to take to school.

The nurse's records must be kept in accordance with the UKCC guidelines for *Standards of Records and Record Keeping*. (See Chapter 2.) Asthma record cards can be purchased from the Asthma Training Centre. The cards act as prompt for the clinic procedure as well as allowing a comprehensive account to be built up of the asthma history and subsequent progress.

Audit

Statistics can be collated about the number of patients on the asthma register, how many of those attended a clinic in the past year, and how many are receiving prophylactic therapy. The number of repeat prescription requests for inhalers can be monitored. If requests are too frequent, or infrequent, the inhalers may not be being used correctly.

Anonymous questionnaires can help in discovering how many patients have asthma symptoms, and how well they comply with the treatment. The reasons for emergency nebulising or hospital admissions can be analysed to see if they could have been prevented by better asthma management.

Diabetes mellitus

A practice with 8000 patients can expect to have about 100 known diabetic patients, but there may be almost as many again undiagnosed. Hence the need for screening.

Diabetes is a chronic metabolic condition caused by a deficiency of insulin, or resistance to its effect; classified as two main types.

Insulin-dependent diabetes mellitus (IDDM)

(Previously called Type I or juvenile onset diabetes.)

This is believed to be an auto-immune condition whereby the islet cells in the pancreas are destroyed, so insulin is not secreted[8]. Children and young adults are most commonly affected.

The treatment is by regular injections of insulin. The aim is to maintain blood glucose levels as near to normal as possible.

Non-insulin dependent diabetes (NIDDM)

(Type II or maturity onset diabetes.)

The cause is still uncertain. NIDDM occurs in later life and is often associated with obesity or a family history of diabetes. Patients of Asian and Afro-Caribbean origin are prone to develop this condition[9].

The treatment may be by diet alone, or diet and hypoglycaemic drugs. NIDDM is not a mild form of diabetes; the complications can be just as serious as those of insulin dependent diabetes, and good blood sugar control is equally important.

Diagnosis

A practice nurse could be the first person to discover that a patient has diabetes; either during routine screening or because the patient has particular risk factors or symptoms. All pregnant women should be screened. Anyone complaining of thirst, polyuria or nocturia; who has recurrent boils or fungal infections, tiredness, paraesthesia, visual changes or ischaemic problems should be tested. A random glucose >11 mmol/l is indicative of diabetes. The patient will need to be referred to the GP, and the education process should be started. In doubtful cases a glucose tolerance test may be requested.

Most patients with IDDM are referred to a diabetologist. The practice policy should determine which group of patients are invited to the diabetic clinic in the practice.

Initial patient education

Most patients will be shocked by the diagnosis of diabetes and will not retain very much information initially. A straightforward explanation about the condition can be backed up by written information to be read at home. A simple diet sheet can be provided, and an appointment made to see a dietician. Patients with polydipsia have often been compounding the problem by drinking gallons of lemonade.

Treatment

Diet

The dietary advice for patients with diabetes does not differ significantly from the sensible eating advised for the rest of the population:

- *Maintain a normal body weight.* Do not consume too many or too few calories.
- *Eat regular meals.*
- *Eat more high fibre starchy foods.* These include: wholemeal bread, wholegrain cereals, jacket potatoes, beans and lentils.
- *Eat less sugar.* Avoid sweets, chocolate, cakes, sugary drinks.
- *Eat less fat.* Cut down on meat and eat more fish and poultry. Have very little butter, cheese and cream; use low fat spreads and skimmed or semi-skimmed milk.
- *Cut down on salt.* Avoid salty foods, use less during cooking, and do not add very much salt to prepared food.
- *Be very careful with alcohol.* Do not exceed the recommended limits for sensible drinking. If overweight, limit the daily consumption to one drink.
- *Do not buy special diabetic foods.* These are unnecessary. Low calorie drinks, artificial sweeteners and tinned fruit in natural juice can be useful[10].

Oral hypoglycaemic agents

Oral hypoglycaemic preparations may be prescribed once it has been shown that dietary restriction alone does not control the blood sugar level[11]. The sulphonylurea drugs (chlorpropramide, glibenclamide, glicazide and tolbutamide) act by stimulating the remaining insulin-secreting cells to perform more efficiently. All these drugs, but particularly chlorpropramide, can occasionally cause hypoglycaemia. They can also cause skin rashes and, on rare occasions, blood disorders.

Metformin (*Glucophage*) acts by increasing the peripheral uptake of glucose. It can be added to the sulphonylurea treatment, or used instead of it.

Insulin

Insulin has to be administered by injection because being a protein it would be digested if given orally. There are many different types of insulin, classified either according to their speed of action, or their source:

- *Short, medium and long-acting insulins.* These can be obtained individually or in various combinations (see *BNF* or *MIMS*).
- *Insulin derived from pork or beef pancreas, or synthetically produced human insulins.* The belief that human insulins prevent the patient recognising the onset of hypoglycaemia have been challenged by research findings[12], but care is needed when changing a patient from one type of insulin to another.

A patient's religious beliefs must be taken into account when prescribing insulin. Jewish and Muslim people cannot use porcine insulin, and Hindus are forbidden to use insulin derived from beef.

Diabetic clinics

The target group may be all patients with diabetes or only non-insulin dependent diabetics. Shared care combines the routine care in the surgery with the management of any difficult problems and/or the annual review, at the hospital unit.

Practice nurse education

The British Diabetic Association (BDA) recommends that nurses who run diabetic clinics should have adequate training[13]; for example the ENB 928 Short Course in Diabetes or equivalent. Diabetes specialist nurses often run updating sessions for practice nurses, and will advise on setting up nurse-run diabetic clinics.

Resources

The *Diabetes Clinical Guidelines for Practice Nurses*[14] provides very comprehensive information and suggests protocols for the minimum, moderate and maximum involvement of nurses in diabetes care. The book also contains details about the specialist diabetes journals and newsletters available. The BDA has published recommendations for diabetes management in primary care[15].

The equipment needed includes:

- scales and a height measure, BMI chart,
- sphygmomanometer and stethoscope,

- urine specimen bottles and test strips,
- phlebotomy equipment.

More specifically:

- blood glucose strips, finger pricking device, lancets and glucose meter,
- Snellen eye chart and pinhole chart for vision testing, mydriatic eye drops (Tropicamide 1%) for preparation for fundoscopy.

Blood glucose meters must be kept clean and calibrated with each batch of test strips. The accuracy of the meter should be tested regularly against a control sample. Finger pricking devices require a new lancet and platform for each patient, to prevent the transmission of blood-borne diseases.

Services

Local social services or district nursing may be required for patients with any disabilities associated with diabetes. A patient with visual problems may need to be referred to the sensory impairment team of the social services; and anyone with impaired mobility may require an occupational therapy assessment. There should be arrangements for prompt access to a dietician and chiropodist.

The British Diabetic Association (BDA) provides information for health professionals as well as for patients. Information about the Association should be given to all diabetic patients. Special holidays can be arranged to teach children to lead a normal life with diabetes.

Procedure for initial consultations

A practice nurse will carry out the tests and investigations specified in the protocol. The initial assessment should cover:

History

- *Social history.* Home situation and family support available, smoking, alcohol, diet and exercise.
- *Occupation and driving.* IDDM precludes some occupations, such as driving heavy goods or public service vehicles. The licensing centre at Swansea must be notified about the diagnosis of diabetes, and the motor insurers should also be informed.

- *Contraception*. A higher dose combined pill may be required if oral hypoglycaemic drugs are used.
- *Medical history*. Previous illnesses and operations.
- *Family history*. History of diabetes, ischaemic conditions, eye problems or hypertension.

Examination

- *Weight, height and BMI*. Patients with IDDM may have lost weight. Patients with NIDDM may be overweight.
- *Urinalysis for:*
    - (a) glucose
    - (b) protein
    - (c) ketones.
- *Blood pressure*. Hypertension increases the risks for CHD and stroke. Hypertension may also be a sign of nephropathy. A postural drop may signify autonomic neuropathy.
- *Feet*. Check the skin condition and circulation, and need for chiropody. Peripheral neuropathy and micro-vascular damage can lead to gangrene if any traumatic lesions or ulcers are not detected early.
- *Eyes*. Check visual acuity with spectacles, if worn.

Blood tests

- *Baseline*. Urea and electrolytes, creatinine, blood glucose, liver function tests, lipids, thyroid function tests.

Education for patients

Discussions should take place to ensure all the staff in general practice and the diabetic unit give consistent information and advice. The amount of information to be given at each visit needs to be judged carefully. Frequent appointments will be required during the initial period of adjustment.

- The patient and family need to understand the reasons for maintaining good blood sugar control, how to monitor the blood sugar levels, and to test the urine for ketones.
- Advice and information are needed on dietary management and how to cope with circumstances such as dinner parties or business lunches.

- A patient stabilised on insulin needs help to master the self-administration of injections.
- Hypoglycaemia must be explained, so the patient knows how to recognise the symptoms and take action to normalise the blood sugar. (See Chapter 7, *Emergency Situations*).
- Patients must know what to do if they are ill. Written instructions can be supplied (Appendix 15.1).
- Preconceptual counselling and close monitoring during pregnancy are essential.
- Ways of coping with travel might need to be discusssed (see Chapter 11).
- A patient whose job is affected may need to be referred for advice to the Disablement Resettlement Officer at the local Job Centre.

Procedure for a routine review:

- Discuss the general health of the patient and any problems experienced.
- Weigh the patient and encourage positive progress towards normal BMI.
- Test urine for glucose, protein, ketones. Send an MSU if any proteinuria is present.
- Screening for microalbuminuria may be carried out using Micro-Bumintest tablets. Persistent microalbuminuria is a predictor for diabetic nephropathy.
- Take a blood sample for glycosylated haemoglobin or fructosamine to check the long-term blood sugar control. (This may be done a week or two before the consultation, so the result is available.)
- Review the results of home blood or urine testing.
- Discuss any problems with the medication or diet.
- Assess the patient's understanding of diabetes and its management. Correct any misunderstandings.
- Teach as required anything the patient is unsure about: the diet, blood glucose monitoring, urinalysis, foot care, insulin injections, hypoglycaemia, coping with illness.

Annual review

In addition to the routine review procedure the annual review should provide a full medical examination, including the feet, injection sites, peripheral pulses and fundi. The diabetic control and treatment should be reviewed. (Blood tests for glucose, HbA1, lipids and creatinine can be taken 2 weeks beforehand, so that the results are ready for the review.)

Patients should be advised that they will be unable to drive for several hours after the pupils have been dilated for fundoscopy. The drops should not be used for patients who have glaucoma or a history of eye surgery. If fundoscopy is not undertaken in the practice, the patient can be examined free of charge by an opthalmic optician.

Records

The practice diabetes register must be kept up-to-date and the patients may also be entered in the district register.

Patients should be encouraged to keep records of their home monitoring and treatment. Patient-held shared care cards allow good communication between the hospital service and the practice. An entry should be made in the patients' records at each encounter.

Defaulters need to be followed up and alternative arrangements suggested if the clinic times are unsuitable. Teenagers can be difficult to help sometimes. Some of them need extra encouragement to take an active part in self-management. Any chronic disease can cause rebellion at this age because the need for conformity with the peer group is so strong. Parents can feel torn by the need to allow them increasing independence if the young people themselves are refusing to take a responsible attitude towards their disease. The natural anxiety for the welfare of their children can make some parents overprotective; thereby increasing the conflict in the home.

Audit

Statistics can be compiled about the patients with diabetes registered with the practice, and compared with the predicted number for the practice size. Details of clinic attendances, waiting times and non-attenders can be collated.

The frequency that certain procedures were carried out: blood pressure measurement, foot checks, blood tests, and eye examinations can be audited.

Other suggestions for audit include: the number of overweight patients who succeeded in losing weight, the levels of glycaemic control achieved, and the number of emergency admissions to hospital. Patient satisfaction can be determined by a questionnaire, and suggestions for improvements to the service can be requested.

Hypertension

High blood pressure increases the risk of heart disease and strokes. The pressure which the blood exerts on the artery walls is created in two main ways: by the *cardiac output* – the force of the blood expelled during systole, and the *peripheral resistance* – the calibre of the arterioles. The blood pressure is controlled centrally from the hypothalamus. Pressure receptors in the aorta and carotid arteries send stimuli to the vasomotor centre, which in turn contols the peripheral resistance via the autonomic nervous system. The cardiac centre controls the rate and contractility of the heart.

The kidneys, which require sufficient pressure for filtration, have their own system for raising the blood presure if it is too low. Renin is secreted by cells near the glomeruli which starts a chain reaction. As a result of which angiotensin II increases the peripheral resistance by vasoconstriction, and stimulates the adrenal cortex to secrete aldosterone, which increases the blood volume through the retention of sodium and water in the renal tubules.

In 80% of patients with high blood pressure, no cause can be established. This is primary or essential hypertension. There may be an inherited tendency, and lifestyle factors can play a part. Secondary hypertension results from another medical condition – neurological, cardiac, renal or endocrine. Hypertension can be life-threatening during pregnancy.

Diagnosis

Blood pressure increases naturally with age and in response to exercise or anxiety. The British Hypertension Society recommends that patients with a persistent BP above 160/90mmHg should be treated[16]. No patient should be diagnosed as hypertensive on one isolated reading. The reading should be repeated on several occasions after resting for at least five minutes.

Treatment

Mild to moderate hypertension may be managed by changes in lifestyle – stopping smoking, increased exercise, reduced alcohol intake, and weight loss if obese. Practice nurses have a particular role in monitoring and encouraging these patients. Medical or surgical treatment may be possible for any condition causing secondary hypertension. Drug therapy is usually required to control more severe hypertension. The drug treatments include:

- *Thiazide diuretics*: e.g. bendrofluazide, may be used alone to control mild hypertension, or in conjunction with other drugs.
- *Beta-blockers*: e.g. atenolol, propranolol, lower blood pressure by reducing the cardiac activity and/or the peripheral resistance, depending on the selectivity of the drug used.
- *Calcium channel blockers*: e.g. nifedipine, diltiazem, prevent the influx of calcium ions across the membrane of smooth muscle, and so reduce vasoconstriction. Some also affect the cardiac output by decreasing the myocardial contractility.
- *Angiotensin-converting enzyme (ACE) inhibiters*: e.g. captopril, enalapril, lisinopril, prevent the conversion of Angiotensin I to Angiotensin II in response to renin secretion; thus preventing peripheral vasoconstriction and aldosterone secretion.

More powerful drugs, hydralazine or prazosin, may be used for patients with severe hypertension which is not controlled by other means.

Hypertension clinics

Nurse education

The training should cover the correct way to measure blood pressure and the maintenance of the equipment, as well as the associated physiology and pharmacology. The training may be obtained through local study days, practice nurse courses, or in-house. It is worth asking a colleague to check a reading sometimes, to see if the results are consistent.

Equipment

Mercury sphygmomanometers are considered to be more reliable for general practice[17]. The manometer needs to stand at 90°, with the mercury levelled at 0. The manometer tube needs to be cleaned regularly; following the manufacturer's instructions. The cuffs should be kept clean. A suede brush is useful for defluffing the velcro fastenings. Cuffs must be available in child's, normal adult and large adult sizes. A thigh cuff is not suitable for an arm. The rubber tubing and balloon should not be perished and the valve must be able to control the release of air at 2mm a second.

Access to a mercury spillage kit is required in case of accidents. (See Chapter 4.)

Protocol

Consensus among general practitioners is not always easy to achieve but there should be a full discussion on when to refer a patient to the GP. The RCN protocol book contains guidelines for hypertension clinics[18]. A standard protocol for hypertension can be used (see Appendix 15.2), but experienced nurses should also be able to use their judgement.

Procedure for a first visit

History

- *Social history*. This includes smoking, alcohol diet and exercise; occupation and stress factors.
- *Medical history*. This includes asthma, diabetes, allergies, heart or kidney disease.
- *Family history*. This includes hypertension, CVS disease, diabetes and renal disease.

Investigations

- *Blood pressure recordings*. The patient should be seated and have rested for ten minutes. Remove restrictive clothing from the arm and position the cuff with the bladder over the brachial artery. The cuff must be on a plane with the patient's heart, and the nurse's angle of view horizontal to the mercury meniscus, for an accurate reading.
- *Height/weight and BMI*. Dietary advice is needed if the patient is overweight.
- *Urinalysis*: for glycosuria and protein.
- *Blood tests*:
    - (a) creatinine, urea and electrolytes for renal function,
    - (b) lipids: to detect hyperlidaemia which increases risks for CHD and stroke,
    - (c) glucose: if diabetes is a possibility.
- *Electrocardiogram*: to show any evidence of left ventricular hypertrophy.

Action

According to the BP and protocol.

Patient education

The education of any patient with a medical condition requires good interpersonal skills. With hypertension in paticular, dire warnings about strokes and heart attacks are more likely to create fear and denial than co-operation. A patient who feels perfectly well must not be turned into a neurotic wreck obsessed with his/her blood pressure readings. Patients need to learn instead about the factors which influence blood pressure and how they can best help themselves to control it.

Procedure for subsequent visits

Enquire about

- Any changes in the patient's general health, lifestyle or social situation since the last visit?
- Any side-effects from the medication (if used) i.e. nausea, diarrhoea, giddiness, lassitude, faintness, impotence, cold extremities?
- Has the patient been taking the drugs (if prescribed)?

Investigations

- Blood pressure: take two readings and calculate the mean pressure.
- Check the patient's weight and calculate the BMI.
- Check the pulse rate (if beta-blockers used).

The nurse must know the blood pressure levels at which she/he is expected to refer the patient back to the doctor.

Education

- Check the patient's understanding of hypertension and any treatment prescribed. Correct any misunderstandings and make sure that the patient is aware of the need to report any side-effects, and not to stop the medication suddenly.
- Encourage appropriate lifestyle changes and praise any successes. (Compliance is more likely if the patient has been given appropriate information and feels in control of the situation[19].)

Records

Hypertension monitoring cards can be kept, or the normal practice record system. A patient-held card is useful if a patient is also being treated at a hospital. It can be infuriating when a patient with well-controlled hypertension has his/her treatment discontinued in hospital because the blood pressure is found to be 'normal'.

The frequency of appointments will depend on the degree of hypertension and its control. The recall system should be able to identify non-attenders, so they do not slip through the net.

Audit

In addition to the clinic statistics an audit may cover:

- The amount by which patients' blood pressures are reduced.
- The incidence of heart attack and stroke in hypertensive patients, with a comparison between those who did, or did not, attend the hypertension clinic.
- The incidence of side-effects with hypotensive drugs.
- Patient satisfaction with the service.

Epilepsy

Epilepsy is described as the tendency to have recurrent seizures. Partial seizures occur when only part of the brain is affected; generalised seizures involve all the brain. Seizures are now classified under these two headings, replacing terms such as: Jacksonian fits, grand mal and petit mal[20].

Partial seizures

These have their onset in a specific part of the brain, although the rest of the brain may subsequently become involved as a generalised seizure.

Simple partial seizures

These cause the sensations of an aura. Consciousness is not impaired, but there may be any variety of sensory, autonomic or psychic symptoms and involuntary movements.

Complex partial seizures

These cause impaired consciousness. This may happen immediately or develop from a simple partial seizure. There may be automatism or odd movements of the mouth.

Generalised seizures

These do not have a focal onset or aura. The two main types are tonic-clonic seizures (previously grand mal) and absences (petit mal).

Tonic-clonic seizures

These have an abrupt onset with a loss of consciousness and bilateraly symmetrical convulsions followed by a period of sleep. (See Chapter 7 for the care of a patient having such a seizure.)

Generalised absences

These are so brief that the patient may be unaware of them. The eyelids may flicker and then consciousness is regained. The patient does not fall down.

Causes

The cause is unknown in most instances. Some epilepsy in childhood may be linked to birth problems or congenital abnormalities, or infections of the nervous system. Tumours or cerebrovascular disease can be a cause of seizures later in life. Trigger factors which can precipitate a seizure include: stress, lack of sleep, alcohol, menstruation, flashing lights, missed tablets.

Diagnosis and treatment

Any patient suspected of having epilepsy should be referred to a neurologist for investigations and decisions about the treatment needed. A history and eye-witness account is needed of the type and frequency of the seizures. The investigations usually include an electro-encephalo-gram (EEG) and magnetic resonance imaging (MRI).

A few localised, accessible lesions may be suitable for neurosurgery but for the majority of patients the seizures will be controlled by drugs. Carbamazepine or sodium valproate are the drugs usually prescribed initially. Others may need to be added in or substituted if the seizures are not controlled. The serum levels of carbamazepine, phenytoin and ethosuximine should be monitored regularly in order to maintain the optimum treatment doses without toxicity.

Epilepsy clinics

The same principles apply to running clinics for patients with epilepsy as they do for the other clinics described above. The aims and target group will need to be identified, and a call/recall system instituted. Practice nurses require education about epilepsy and a protocol for a nurse-run clinic. Epilepsy liaison nurses are currently visiting practices around the country to help nurses to learn how to provide a service comparable to that for patients with asthma and diabetes.

Audit

Whatever practice nurses undertake in the field of heath promotion for patients with chronic diseases, the requirement to produce evidence of its worth remains. In fact the greater the number of opportunities for nurse involvement, the greater the need to use the scarce resources most effectively. Which means finding ways to ensure that the aims of the health promotion activities are being fulfilled.

Suggestions for evaluation and research

- Devise a study to discover how many patients with prescribed metered dose inhalers are able to use them correctly.
- Devise a study of patients diagnosed as diabetic within the past five years to find out:
    - (a) what help the patients received from nurses, when they were newly diagnosed,
    - (b) what help they would like to have received,
    - (c) what changes you might make to your nursing practice.
- Conduct a literature search on the effectiveness of nurse-run hypertension clinics in general practice.
- Review your practice population profile and note the prevalence of particular chronic diseases in the locality. Prepare a report on ways that the primary health care team could work together to improve the service offered to patients with those conditions.

References

1. RCN Issues in Nursing and Health Initiatives (1988) Protocols: guidance for good practice; *Nursing Standard*, **8**(8): 29.
2. Parliamentary Office of Science and Technology (1994) *Breathing in Our Cities*. PO of S&T, London.
3. Asthma Training Centre (1990) *Distance Learning Package*, Unit 1: 2. ATC, Stratford-upon-Avon.
4. Day, M. (1993) New thinking on asthma management; *Practice Nurse*, **5**: 933–936, 942.

5. British Medical Association and Royal Pharmaceutical Society of Great Britain (1993) *British National Formulary.* 112.
6. Walters, O. and Pederson, S. (1993) Short-term growth during treatment with inhaled fluticasone proprionate and beclamethasone diproprionate; *Archive of Disease in Childhood,* **68:** 673–676.
7. Smail, J. *Protocols for Health Promotion Clinics,* RCN and South Glamorgan FHSA.
8. Cradock, S. (1993) Non-insulin dependent diabetes; *Primary Health Care,* **3**(5): 16.
9. Bower, H. (1993) Seeing health in black and white; *Practice Nurse,* **6:** 616.
10. British Diabetic Association *Dietary Recommendations – A Basic Guide,* BDA, London.
11. British Medical Association, Royal Pharmaceutical Society of Great Britain (1993) *British National Formulary.* 254.
12. News (1993) Hypos unaffected by insulin type; *Practice Nurse,* **6:** 9.
13. British Diabetic Association (1987, revised 1991) *Minimal Educational Requirements for the Care of Diabetes in the UK,* BDA, London.
14. Royal College of Nursing (1992) *Diabetes Clinical Guidelines for Practice Nurses,* printed by Bayer Diagnostics.
15. Diabetes Services Advisory Committee, British Diabetic Association (1993) *Recommendations for the Management of Diabetes in Primary Care.* BDA, London.
16. Sever, P., Beevers, G., Bulpitt, C., Lever, A., Ramsay, L., Reid, J. and Swales, J. (1993) Management guidelines in essential hypertension: report of the second working party of the British Hypertension Society; *British Medical Journal,* **306:** 983–987.
17. Beevers, D.G. and Macgregor, G.A. (1987) *Hypertension in Practice.* 71–72. Martin Dunitz, London.
18. Smail, J. *Protocols for Health Promotion Clinics.* RCN and South Glamorgan FHSA.
19. Cameron, K. and Gregor, F. (1987) Chronic illness and compliance; *Journal of Advanced Nursing,* **12:** 671–676.
20. Taylor, M. (1990) Epilepsy and its diagnosis; *Practice Nurse,* **3:** 29–31.

Further reading

Tettersell, M.J. (1993) Asthma patients' knowledge in relation to compliance with drug therapy; *Journal of Advanced Nursing,* **18:** 103–113.

Useful addresses

Asthma Training Centre
Winton House,
Church Street,
Stratford-upon-Avon, CV37 6HB.
Telephone 0789-296974 *Fax* 0789-261027.

National Asthma Campaign
300 Upper Street, London N1 2XX.
Telephone 071-226 2260 *Fax* 071-704 0740.

British Diabetic Association
10 Queen Anne Street,
London W1M 0BD.
Telephone 071-323 1531.

British Epilepsy Association
Anstey House,
40 Hanover Square,
Leeds LS3 1BD.
Telephone 0532-439393.

National Society for Epilepsy
Chalfont Centre for Epilepsy,
Chalfont St Peter,
Gerrards Cross,
Bucks SL9 0RT.

Epilepsy Association of Scotland
48 Govan Road,
Glasgow G51 1JR.

Appendix 15.1
Guidelines for patients with diabetes on coping with sickness

If you are unwell, or have a gastric upset, your diabetes is likely to be affected. The following guidelines should be followed:

(1) Do not stop your insulin even if you do not feel like eating. (Consult your doctor if on oral treatment – the dose may need to be reduced.)
(2) Check your diabetes control at least four times a day (blood or urine test).
(3) Have plenty of sugar-free drinks to prevent yourself becoming dehydrated.
(4) Test your urine for ketones.
(5) If unable to eat your normal meals take measured small amounts (10–20g) of concentrated carbohydrates every hour e.g.:
    30ml non-diet Ribena
    50ml Lucozade
    100ml natural unsweetened fruit juice
    100ml non-diet coke
    200ml milk.
(6) Consult your doctor if:
    (a) unable to keep fluids down,
    (b) there are large amounts of ketones in your urine,
    (c) your blood sugar control remains unstable.

Appendix 15.2
Blood pressure protocol for nurses

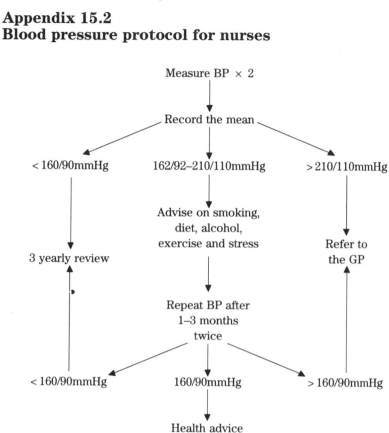

Measure BP × 2

Record the mean

< 160/90mmHg   162/92–210/110mmHg   > 210/110mmHg

Advise on smoking,
diet, alcohol,
exercise and stress

Refer to
the GP

3 yearly review

Repeat BP after
1–3 months
twice

< 160/90mmHg   160/90mmHg   > 160/90mmHg

Health advice

Annual review

Conclusion

Writing a text book can seem like observing the countryside throughout the seasons – the landscape keeps changing.

Research findings in medicine and nursing can turn the accepted wisdom upside-down in a moment. Every week new developments seem to occur, about which patients may learn from television or the radio long before the official directives reach general practice. All of this goes to show how important it is to keep an open mind and be willing to challenge everything.

According to Plato, the philosopher Socrates, when asked about the source of his wisdom, maintained that he knew nothing, and was only wiser than others in knowing that he knew nothing. I used to find that rather puzzling, but now it seems strangely comforting. It means that we should never stop enquiring, and searching for knowledge.

This book does not profess to supply all the answers, but hopefully the readers will have a better idea of the questions.

G.D.H

Index